I'M EXPECTIN

YOUR STEP-BY-STEP GUIDE FOR ANTENATAL &
HYPNOBIRTHING PREPARATION

JACKIE KIETZ

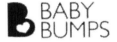

Dedication

A big thank you to all those who helped with the book by reading through it and reviewing it – I am very grateful.

All the love to my family as without you, writing this book would not have been possible.

Note to readers

This book and the techniques and information within it are not intended to replace medical care from qualified healthcare professionals. It is a guide to your options and choices, enabling you to discuss your wishes in detail with your midwife/doctor. The author and publisher cannot accept responsibility for readers' personal decisions about which techniques and information they use during birth.

The book is aimed at women with straightforward pregnancies. Women with more complex needs during pregnancy may find that they have a different balance of benefits and risks than women with straightforward pregnancies.

Please note that illustrations are for general information and are not anatomically precise.

Whilst the author trained with the National Childbirth Trust (NCT) this book is in no way affiliated, authorised or endorsed by the NCT.

About the author

Jackie Kietz trained with and facilitates antenatal courses for the National Childbirth Trust (NCT). She is a hypnobirthing practitioner and founder of Baby Bumps Hypnobirthing in South East London. In addition she is a baby massage instructor and reflexologist specialising in maternity reflexology and BabyReflex classes for parents.

For more information visit www.baby-bumps.net.

Contents

Foreword

If you are looking for a book that offers you clear, readable information about your birth, then look no further. Jackie's guide covers all the subjects you will want to consider as you prepare for the day of your baby's arrival.

She combines a wealth of knowledge and experience of pregnancy and birth with a direct writing style. The book is an easy, informative read that will prepare you for making choices about your care and how you would like your birth to be. If you want to do more detailed research of your own, the references provided will keep you busy.

I recommend this book to all expectant parents.

Mark Harris, midwife and author of Men, Love & Birth (Pinter and Martin, 2015)

Preface

A very warm welcome to you, reader!

This book has been written for pregnant women and their birth partners. The guidelines discussed are UK-based and are just that – guidelines. In the UK maternity units' guidelines vary from Trust to Trust, and policies and guidelines may change or be amended

The aim of the book is to give you a good, general overview of your choices and options for labour and birth where you will not find any unexplained jargon. It is a starting point for your thinking about what you might like for your birth and it can also act as a recap of any antenatal course you may have done. You can use it as a quick reference guide or reminder of your options.

Some women are not aware that they have choices about how their labour and birth unfolds. Whilst no one can predict how a birth may go, this guide talks you through what some of your options may be. Most chapters have references and suggested further reading, and there are more links at the end of the book too, so you can research for yourself and go on to have informed discussions with your midwife about your care.

I wish you all the very best on your amazing journey!

Jackie Kietz, September 2016

Introduction

In my capacity as an antenatal and hypnobirthing practitioner, I often meet expectant parents who are unaware they have choices. All too often I hear 'Am I allowed?', or say 'I was told I had to...'. I have written this guide as a simple introduction to the possible choices and options available to parents during their baby's birth, and hope that it will help you as you prepare for the birth of your baby.

Having a baby and becoming a mother or a father is, of course, a life-changing experience. The circumstances of the birth, and how women and their partners feel as it unfolds, can have long-lasting effects: ask any parent about their memories of their children's births and you will usually find that they remember it in detail and how they felt during and after it, whether positive or negative.

I know that not everyone can afford to attend private antenatal classes, where parents have the luxury of time to go through all the options available during labour and birth. Although there is a lot of information available in books, magazines and on the internet, it's not easy to find clear and simple discussion of birth choices.

Sometimes during birth there are decisions to be made, and this book outlines the benefits and risks for typical decisions that may need to be made during 'low-risk' pregnancies/labours so you can then discuss these with your caregivers should you wish to.

Unlike many labour and birth books, this book is an all-round guide that covers traditional medical and non-medical options for managing labour and birth. So as well as being informed about medical interventions, you will also cover hypnobirthing and the power of the mind to affect labour and birth, with hypnobirthing scripts and MP3 downloads included in your purchase of this book.

The book talks through the process of labour from the start to the end. It gives practical suggestions to mothers and birth partners on how to get the most comfortable birth possible, what can hinder this, and what they can do about it.

References/further reading and websites are listed for those interested.

1

THE STAGES OF LABOUR AND WHAT TO EXPECT

Throughout this book I may refer to 'contractions' as 'surges' – this is just a different way to describe the work of the uterus. You may hear both terms used during your pregnancy and labour. The labour I describe below is a 'textbook' labour. As all women are different, many will find that their pattern of labour varies. Typically labour is divided into three stages – but this may be more for record-keeping than anything else, and labour is often not as clearly defined as the stages suggest! However, you will probably hear the three stages mentioned during your pregnancy and in labour, so in this chapter we go through each one in turn.

You have probably heard of dilation of the cervix, or the cervix needing to open from 0cm to 10cm. The cervix is found internally – it is at the top of the vagina/birth canal and is the opening to the uterus, or the neck of the womb. During pregnancy, a woman's cervix is normally closed and has a mucus plug in it to keep out infection, which is called a 'show' when it comes away. Before dilation starts the cervix is around 3cm long, firm and points slightly towards the woman's back.

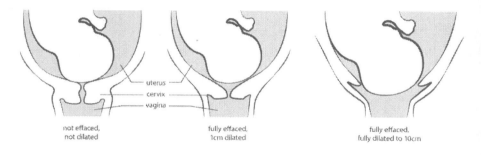

not effaced,
not dilated

fully effaced,
1cm dilated

fully effaced,
fully dilated to 10cm

1.) The cervix is thick, long and firm. In preparation for the start of labour the cervix first needs to move from a posterior position (pointing towards your back) to an anterior position, so it is pointing more towards your front. Then it needs to shorten and soften, which is sometimes referred to as 'ripening'.

This ripening can start in late pregnancy before labour has started, or in early labour. Some women notice the mucus plug coming away (the show). It is a mucous-like looking discharge and as it is mixed with blood it is usually pinky or a bit bloody. This is not a sign that labour is imminent, but it is a sign that the body is getting ready and the cervix is starting to soften and open.

2.) As you can see, the cervix in image 2 is fully effaced (thinned out) and has started to open (dilate). This is what your surges do – the strong muscular work of the surges draws the cervix up into the body of the uterus and it becomes thinner and then opens.

3.) Image 3 shows a fully dilated cervix. As the cervix is internal, at the top of the vagina, you will not know how dilated you are unless you examine yourself or a midwife does this for you. Sometimes women know instinctively how far along in their labour they are, and sometimes a midwife can tell by closely observing a woman's behaviour. If women have practised hypnobirthing, they can often appear very calm late on in their labours, which may mean that those caring for them underestimate how well and far on labour has progressed. Therefore it is important to tell your midwife if you are using hypnobirthing techniques.

Signs that your body is getting ready for labour (pre-labour):

- Increased practice contractions, or 'Braxton Hicks' contractions. Many women find these painless and are sometimes unaware they're having them, or they may notice their bump go hard and tight for a moment. Other women feel them strongly or get a period pain type sensation with them. Sometimes women have runs of Braxton Hicks contractions in the evenings for several days before the process of labour starts.

- Backache, or a pre-menstrual feeling.

- Waters releasing – this can be a gush or a trickle and can sometimes occur before labour starts or during it. You should let your maternity unit know when your waters have released.

- A show – the mucous plug can sometimes come away.

- The start of surges.

- Feeling different: maybe feeling restless, irritable or not sleeping well.

- An upset stomach, diarrhoea or a frequent need to open your bowels. This is caused by changes in the level of certain hormones your body released before labour starts. Don't worry about this – it is positive - the body is making as much room as possible for your baby's journey out.

- Nesting instinct – an urge to get your home in order and everything ready.

- 'Lightening' – this is the term to describe the baby's head moving into your pelvis. Women usually feel that they can breathe more easily after this, as when the baby 'drops' there is more room for the woman's lungs. This often happens a few weeks before labour starts.

As there can be an overlap between pre-labour and the start of labour itself, you may find it hard to tell whether or not labour has really started.

What do contractions feel like?

This varies from woman to woman. Some women feel them strongly and others just feel a tightening sensation.

Contractions can be felt in the groin, lower abdomen and sometimes down the tops of the legs. Some women feel uncomfortable around their bump and back, or experience a heavy feeling low down in their pelvis. Typically, contractions start off short and mild, with long gaps in between each one, and as labour progresses the contractions get longer, stronger and closer together.

When labour starts – the first stage

The first stage of labour includes 'early labour' and 'active labour'. As a rough guide, early labour is when surges are opening the cervix from 0–4cm, and the active stage of labour is when the cervix is opening from 4–10cm.

Early labour

During this stage surges are usually (though not always) irregular, perhaps coming every 15–20 minutes and lasting around 20-30 seconds. They may peter out, then start up again.

Labour can start at any time of the day or night. It often starts at night when you feel safe, secure - and it's dark and warm in bed. Your brain thinks 'Ah, this is a good, safe time to go into labour!' As exciting as it is, try to go back to sleep (or at least rest if it's the middle of the night); your body will be grateful for the rest. Putting on one of the hypnobirthing MP3s may help.

How can you help yourself in early labour?

- Have a bath.

- Eat! Go with what you fancy, but high-fat foods may make you feel sick and your digestive system needs to rest. Not eating in labour can lead to a woman feeling tired and weak later on, which can lead to unnecessary interventions. You could try toast, cereal, pasta, soup or sandwiches. Stay hydrated too.

- It may sound crazy, but distractions such as baking a cake or making a dish you haven't done before are useful, as you're focused on the recipe, you're upright and moving around which helps labour along, and you'll have a lovely meal or cake to enjoy once your baby has arrived. Remember, contractions are usually mild in early labour so it's quite possible you could manage to do this if it's of interest.

- Go for a local, relaxing walk.

- Rest with a book.

- Try to sleep.

- Watch or listen to comedy or a light-hearted box set – not only is this distracting, but laughter is also relaxing and produces feel-good hormones such as oxytocin and endorphins, which help keep labour progressing beautifully.

- If you are using a TENS machine, you can put it on in early labour. (A TENS machine is a form of pain management which we cover later).

The first stage of labour is usually the longest, but varies hugely from woman to woman. For first-time mothers it can be anything from 8 and 20+ hours, with subsequent births often being quicker. The hormones released during labour distort your perception of time, so labour doesn't always necessarily feel as long as it is.

Staying at home during this stage has many benefits, one of which is that a familiar and relaxing environment helps labour progress smoothly. At home you can get into your own groove more easily, as it's your territory and you have all your home comforts around you. You can eat and drink what & when you like, rest in your own bed & come and go as you please.

You can call the labour ward as many times as you like during this stage to seek reassurance from a midwife, who will be happy to answer any questions you have.

Active labour

In active labour your surges become longer, stronger, closer together and of increased intensity, each one requiring all of your attention and focus. As a rough guide, surges will be come around every 3 minutes, last about 1 minute, and will have been doing this for at least an hour. But do remember that we are talking about a textbook labour! All women experience labour differently, with some starting off with regular, strong surges and others never getting into a regular pattern.

During this stage tune into your body and how you are feeling. If you no longer want to chat through your surges, but instead want to stop what you're doing, turn your focus inwards and use deep breathing to help you, then you are most probably in active labour.

You may feel hot, and may not be interested in eating or talking much. You may also start to feel less inhibited, which is great as you are then able to follow your body's lead.

The intensity of the surges encourages you to move and get into one or many of the positions you will have practised during your pregnancy (more on positions for labour later). Following your body's lead and moving, rocking and swaying makes labour feel more manageable and helps your baby get into a good position, as well as increasing the release of some of the fantastic birthing hormones.

If you are planning a birth in hospital or at a birth centre (see the chapter Place of Birth), then this is the time to get ready to go in. If you are planning a homebirth, let your home birth midwife know that you feel you are in active labour.

When you call to say you feel that you are in active labour and would like to come in to the labour ward/birth centre, the midwife may want to speak with you during several contractions as part of the assessment to try to gauge how you are responding to them. She will also want to get a bit of background information from your partner.

As mentioned before, if you have prepared using hypnobirthing always let the midwife know, as you will likely appear calmer than expected for a woman in active labour. Trust your body and what you are feeling rather than how you are expected to be behaving.

How can you help yourself during active labour?

If you have not already started to focus on your breathing, now is the time. Slow, deep, calming breathing, with the 'out' breath a little longer than the 'in' breath, will help to keep you relaxed and focused as you leave home to transfer into hospital.

- Slow, deep, calm breathing will save energy and bring you and your baby increased oxygen, helping your uterus do its incredible job.

- Massage from your birth partner may be beneficial, though some women prefer not to be touched during active labour.

- Staying hydrated and eating what you fancy.

- Emptying your bladder regularly – an empty bladder creates more space for your baby. Your birth partner can remind you to do these things.

Take one surge at a time and continue breathing deeply until you reach the end of the first stage, which is usually signalled by the changing sensations and a feeling of pressure in the back passage, which is followed by an urge to bear down or push. This is called the second stage of labour, or the pushing or breathing down stage.

Sometimes women have a lull in contractions before the second stage starts and can rest a little.

Vaginal examinations

Vaginal examinations are usually offered at around four-hourly intervals once active labour has started, as part of assessing the woman's progress. Your consent should always be given before any intervention takes place. They are sometimes offered on arrival at hospital, or when your home birth midwife arrives. If you wish, you can request one.

Sometimes a woman may choose not to have any examinations, as they find them invasive and uncomfortable. Some women prefer not to know how many centimetres they are dilated and instead be guided by their own bodies.

You can choose to accept one initial vaginal examination and then decline any others, or you can agree to have examinations as offered. It is always your choice whether you consent to an examination, or not, and you do not necessarily have to be laying flat on the bed to have one done, for example you may be in a different position in the pool.

Examinations offer a 'screen shot' of that moment and knowing the dilation of the cervix will not predict when a woman will give birth. Some women can progress very quickly if the environment is right and they feel safe and secure. If a woman becomes anxious or unable to relax her labour may slow down and she may pause at, for example, 6cm, if in her mind she is unable to let go.

Sometimes a midwife may inadvertently break the waters during an examination. Waters are the amniotic fluid that surrounds the baby. The waters act as a cushion between the baby's head and the woman's cervix, and when they release this cushioning disappears, which can make surges feel more intense.

Once the waters have released this puts a bit of clock watch on progression meaning that if labour does not progress within certain parameters after this point, other interventions will be offered to augment (speed up) the labour. These which come with their own set of risks (and which you can ask questions about before deciding to accept or decline)

Second stage

The second stage of labour starts when the cervix has fully dilated and ends when the baby is born. It can be very short, or as long as 3 hours, for a first-time mother.

The start of the second stage of labour is the journey the baby takes through the vagina (or some call it birth canal) to the outside world. Surges are usually intense and expulsive, lasting about 1-1.5 minutes long as the powerful uterus nudges him down and out of your vagina. Many like it to the sensation of opening the bowels, which like contractions, are an involuntary process when the mother feels safe and birth is allowed to unfold in its own way.

Breathing and positions for the second ('pushing' or 'nudging your baby down') stage

There is more later on in the book on breathing techniques, but during surges it is important to continue deep breathing, bringing valuable oxygen to your baby and uterus. So rather than holding your breath and pushing hard against your body, work with your body and follow its lead. It knows what it is doing.

It can help to take a deep breath in through your nose (or mouth if you have a blocked nose) and then, with your mouth closed and jaw relaxed, breathe out firmly but gently, sending the breath out through your nose and down towards your pelvic floor, giving your baby a helpful nudge downwards when the urge to push is felt.

You may want to repeat this breathing technique 3–5 times during the longer, expulsive second-stage surges. Each oxygen-fuelled, powerful breath will help your baby on his journey down. Resisting holding your breath and pushing hard against your body may help to prevent tearing.

Move around and change position as your body dictates. You may like to try not to lie flat, or semi-flat (you can read more about useful labour and birth positions later in the book). Remember to empty your bladder regularly, particularly if your breathing down/pushing efforts are ineffective.

How you can help yourself during second stage

- Maintain long, deep, powerful breaths, which focus downwards, helping your baby on his journey into the world.

- Consider which positions you can adopt that will create room in your pelvis.

- If you are concerned about opening your bowels at this stage, you can sit on the toilet or straddle the toilet and lean over on the cistern (put a pillow on it) – this is safe to do and a great position to be in. Don't worry, you won't have your baby in the toilet! You will know when your baby's almost ready to be born and will have moved by this point.

- Having sips of coconut water, or a healthy alternative, to replace lost electrolytes can help boost energy. It's important to keep hydrated throughout your labour.

- Again, remember to empty your bladder regularly.

- Know that each powerful surge is bringing you closer to finally meeting your baby!

Further reading

Signs that labour has begun. NHS Choices, Health A-Z. NHS. 2015. www.nhs.uk (Accessed August 2016)

Early signs of labour. NCT. 2015. www.nct.org.uk (Accessed August 2016)

Intrapartum care for healthy women and babies. NICE guidelines [CG190], NICE, 2014. www.nice.org.uk (Accessed August 2016)

Downe S, Gyte GML, Dahlen HG, Singata M, *Routine vaginal examinations in labour*, 2013. www.cochrane.org/CD010088/routine-vaginal-examinations-in-labour (accessed September 2016)

Nutrition in labour. Evidence based guidelines for midwifery-led care in labour. Royal College of Midwives, 2012. www.rcm.org.uk (Accessed August 2016)

I'M EXPECTING A BABY

THE THIRD STAGE – DELIVERY OF THE PLACENTA

This is the stage from when your baby is born until the placenta (sometimes called afterbirth) is birthed and any bleeding is under control. After you have had your baby contractions will continue so the body starts the process of releasing the placenta. As it is a soft organ, it is easier to birth. Holding your baby skin to skin and if you're planning on breastfeeding doing this during this stage. Skin to skin and breastfeeding can help with the third stage as both these things produce the hormone oxytocin which helps with the safe delivery of the placenta.

There are two types of third stage and you can think about what you would prefer now, or at the time. How your birth has gone may impact your decision around this.

Active management

This is made up of three components. You are given an injection in the thigh that helps the uterus to contract strongly, the cord is clamped and cut after 1–5 minutes and the midwife carefully pulls the placenta out via the cord while supporting your uterus externally with her hand – this is called controlled cord traction. Active management shortens the third stage, and there is some evidence that it reduces the risk of heavy bleeding. It increases the chance of nausea and vomiting and causes a slight increase in blood pressure.

Physiological management

This means there is no intervention. The mother holds her baby while he is still attached by the umbilical cord to the placenta.

During a physiological third stage the cord is not clamped and cut - either until it stops pulsating (this 'pulsating' is the baby's blood moving from the placenta & cord into the baby) or until the placenta is delivered - so the baby gets his full quota of blood and the placenta is delivered by maternal effort. There is a slightly higher chance of heavy bleeding with a physiological third stage.

Why might a woman opt for a physiological third stage?

During the third stage the placenta starts to come away from the wall of the uterus and then it is moved down into the vagina by contractions where it is birthed.

Around a third of the baby's blood is inside the cord and placenta at any one time. If the cord is clamped and cut straight away, this blood that is rich in iron and stem cells, is not passed to its rightful owner – the baby.

By waiting around 10 minutes before clamping and cutting the cord, the oxygenated blood from the placenta and cord will have passed into the baby. This means he will have good iron stores and enough blood to fill all the vessels around his lungs, making breathing easier for that first breath. With this way of delivering the placenta the cord is usually clamped and cut after the placenta has been delivered, or when the cord has stopped pulsating.

Why might a woman want to have an actively managed third stage?

Sometimes it may be safer for a woman to have active management of the third stage. If there is heavy bleeding, if the birth has been very long, complicated or medically managed — for example, if she has needed an induction of labour (when labour is started using drugs) or augmentation of labour (when labour is speeded up using drugs), or if she has had an assisted birth (using forceps or ventouse) — an active third stage is safer as the risk of having heavy blood loss increases when things are less straightforward.

You can make a decision about how you want to have the third stage in advance and then see how the birth progresses. You could start off with a planned physiological third stage and then opt for the injection at any point, or you can choose active management. It may also be possible to have delayed cord clamping at a caesarean birth, though this would need to be discussed in advance.

You can always change your mind about your choices and talk to your midwife about it at the time. If you do opt for a managed third stage, you can usually wait up to 5 minutes before the cord is clamped and cut, meaning your baby will receive the majority of his blood.

How can you help yourself during the third stage?

- Hold your baby skin-to-skin (her bare skin against your bare skin).

- Breastfeed your baby, if this is something you are planning to do.

- There is some evidence that when women have skin to skin contact with their baby after birth and breastfeed them there are fewer postpartum haemorrhages (PPH).

- Adopt an upright position to utilise gravity's force – kneeling on the bed is a good position.

- Keep the lights low.

- Keep warm – some women are shivery after birth, due to the increased adrenalin. Increased adrenalin can slow the third stage down. Have your partner put a blanket around you.

- Empty your bladder – a full bladder can slow the third stage down.

References & further reading

Information for the public. Delivering the Placenta, NICE. www.nice.org.uk (Accessed August 2016)

Saxton, A, Fahy, K & Hastie, C. *Effects of skin-to-skin contact and breastfeeding at birth on the incidence of PPH: A physiologically based theory.* 2015. www.researchgate.net (Accessed September 2016)

Intrapartum care for healthy women and babies. NICE guidelines [CG190], NICE, 2014. www.nice.org.uk (Accessed August 2016)

Third Stage of Labour. NCT. www.nct.org.uk (Accessed August 2016)

STAY AT HOME OR CALL AND GO IN?

You should call the labour ward if:

- You experience reduced movements. This is important throughout your pregnancy as well as during your labour. Movements should not lessen or slow down the bigger your baby gets — there will not be any 'somersaults' in the later weeks of pregnancy due to the lack of room, but the *amount* of movements you feel should be the same as before. Babies' movements do not slow down as pregnancy progresses.

- You have any fluid loss, or you think your waters may have released. Waters should be clear — if they are tinged with brown or green, or have any strong odour, you should go in and get this checked out. It may mean your baby needs monitoring.

- You have any blood loss.

- You have a headache or visual disturbances such as colours, patches or blurred vision.

- You have sudden swelling of the face and hands

- You have a rash, or itching.

- You are in any constant abdominal pain or have pain passing urine.

- You have a raised temperature or you just do not feel 'right'.

- You have any concerns whatsoever. If you do, call the labour ward. They are there for you and you are not wasting their time. Don't be fobbed off if you feel something is not right. Call as many times as you need to and never put things off or wait to see how you or your baby are the following day.

Going in

It can sometimes be hard antenatally to understand how you will know when you are in labour and how you will know when to transfer in.

As discussed in chapter 1, there may be a time where you are wondering 'Is this it, has my labour started for real?' You may wonder if you are just having more Braxton Hicks contractions.

Usually, it becomes obvious that you are in labour, as the surges get closer together, longer and stronger and take all of your attention to manage. You no longer want to chat through them, but want to turn your focus inwards and breathe through them.

If things are ticking along and you are having a straightforward pregnancy, staying at home as long as possible has many benefits, such as:

- It's your familiar environment, where you feel relaxed.

- You can eat and drink whatever you want; no need to get hot drinks from a machine!

- You can have a bath or shower in your own space.

- You can rest in your own familiar and comforting bed.

- You can watch a comedy box set or something that makes you relax and laugh while moving and bouncing on your birth ball – distractions are so useful!

- You have everything at home that you need and it is the best place to be for early labour.

- Research shows that staying at home in early labour means it progresses more efficiently.

Most women want to transfer in or ask their home birth midwife to come over when contractions have been coming every 3minutes, lasting about a minute and have been like this for at least an hour. Typically, this is how surges will feel in active labour, though we are of course all wonderfully different.

Still unsure? In the absence of a history of precipitate (very fast) labours, if you find yourself wondering whether it's time to go in or you are still chatting through surges, it is probably too early. It could mean that just a short while after you turn to your partner and say 'I want to go in — now!', but any time before that you really are better off nesting at home.

The journey in

It is quite common for labour to slow down or completely stall when women leave their familiar nest and go into the relative unknown. As well as feeling excited, you may feel a little anxious, which is perfectly understandable.

Anxiety increases adrenalin levels in the body, which can hinder labour. We are the same as our mammal friends — if a labouring animal notices a predator, feels anxious, or out of her safe place (home, for us humans), her adrenalin levels rise and pause her labour. She will attempt to find a safe place to hide until the threat goes away, and her labour will restart when she feels relaxed. We are the same — but luckily we don't have any predators lurking!

To help with the transition from home to your chosen place of birth, it is well worth doing a tour of the birth centre/hospital beforehand, so it is familiar to you and you know what the parking situation is. Get rid of as many 'unknowns' as possible in advance.

Some hospitals have large car parks with a section dedicated to maternity. Others are very tight for space, especially in London, and have parking restrictions at certain times of the day in the surrounding roads. Doing your homework first is helpful. Not all hospitals offer a tour and instead there is an online tour.

Many women choose to take a taxi instead, and of course not everyone has access to a car. If you are planning on taking a taxi ring around and find around three different cab companies that are willing to take a woman in labour, as not all do. Your local hospital may be able to recommend taxi companies that will take labouring women. You can explain that you will bring a towel to sit on (the usual concern is about waters leaking into their upholstery!).

If you own a car, your partner can then get a cab home after the birth and come and pick you up in your own car, with your car seat ready to take your precious cargo home.

Another option is to draft in a family member or friend to be on call to take you to hospital.

How can you help yourself when transferring from home

- Visit your chosen place of birth in advance.

- Assuming all has been well in your pregnancy, try not to be tempted to go in too early — wait until your contractions are strong, long and close together.

- Try to keep 'in the zone' by blocking out external noise and light.

- You can plug in your headphones and listen to music or your hypnobirthing /relaxation MP3. Or use earplugs to block out the world and keep your focus inwards.

- Put on an eye mask or sunglasses in the taxi.

- Cover up with a big hoody.

- Try your best to keep your senses turned inwards and ask your partner to deal with the admin and questions.

- Don't worry about how you look — you'll probably never see any of these people again!

Keep this going until you get into your labour room or birth centre, and then you can adjust the room as you see fit to make it cosy and dark.

4

HORMONES AND ENVIRONMENT – WHAT HELPS AND HINDERS LABOUR?

When the long-awaited day finally comes around and you begin to give birth to a tiny, *brand new human being* you will be at your most powerful! A woman in labour is an incredible force – but she is also vulnerable. Her senses will be heightened and how she is feeling and her immediate environment will have a huge impact on how her well her labour progresses.

To help things go super smoothly, you need to feel safe, secure, warm and – most importantly – undisturbed. Ideally you won't be 'watched over', or unduly interrupted or questioned. As birth is pretty primal, you want the rational, logical, thinking part of your brain well and truly out of the picture so you can get into your own private zone.

Even small things can tip you out of this undisturbed state and into feeling anxious, and your immediate environment can play a big part. Giving birth is the most private and personal thing you will ever do – along with getting intimate with your significant other – and of course the two are intrinsically linked. You need to create a similar environment for birth as you would when making love. Usually for most this would be an environment with low lighting, not having people wandering in and out, not having someone asking us how we are progressing and 'can we hurry up a bit', not having someone make suggestions on how we should be 'doing it' and not being told what position we should be in. Can you imagine this happening when you're getting cosy with your partner! Nothing would be more likely to shut your body down, clamp it up and cause everything to stall; it's the same for birth.

Think of when you have watched an animal give birth on a wildlife documentary. She will give birth when she feels safe, usually hidden away and in the dark. She will appear calm and relaxed and will use movement and low, quiet sounds to help her. If she feels threatened, she will halt her labour until she feels safe again.

We fellow mammals need the same quiet, dark, private conditions to give birth well and feeling observed, fearful or anxious will have a very real effect on the progress of labour. Interruptions, (usually) giving birth in a public building, bright lights, being poked and prodded by a relative stranger and potentially being told to 'hurry up or we'll need to intervene' are all a huge hindrance and take a woman out of her all important private birthing zone. Without going into great detail about birthing hormones, I do want to explain them briefly how they are affected by environment.

Oxytocin is the powerhouse hormone of labour. We don't know exactly what starts labour, but oxytocin is one hormone that shapes the length and strength of surges. Released in pulses, it helps the muscles of the uterus contract to gently open the cervix. This muscular contraction signals the brain to produce more oxytocin, keeping labour beautifully effective and rhythmic. It is also known as the 'hormone of love', because amongst other things, it is released when couples make love, and when people feel relaxed, happy, safe and secure. It comes out in abundance when it is dark (the hormone melatonin helps with that) and coupled with high levels of endorphins will help to make labour feel more comfortable and keeps the woman feeling calm.

The fight-or-flight hormones, adrenaline and noradrenaline, are produced by the body in response to stresses such as hunger, fear/anxiety and cold. When these hormones kick in, our body gets ready to 'freeze, fight or flight'.

It is normal for there to be adrenalin during the transition part of labour (towards the end of the first stage) and when the uterus is nudging the baby out. However, if a woman has high levels of adrenalin during her whole labour it can inhibit her contractions, slowing or even stopping labour. Blood flow to the uterus and placenta is reduced, which not only affects labour and comfort levels, but can also affect the baby.

'Fight or flight' is a great tool for emergency, life-or-death situations and for wild animals giving birth, as this reflex inhibits labour and sends blood to the major muscle groups, so the birthing mother can most likely choose to flee from a threat. We are lucky enough not to have such threats when we give birth, but as already mentioned, bright lights, feeling as if we are being observed, frequent interruptions and feeling fearful and anxious can quite easily tip a woman into this state. As a result, surges are less efficient, more painful and labour may slow or even stop completely.

Beta-endorphin

These are naturally occurring opiates which are our very own, in-house, powerful painkillers with similar properties to morphine and pethidine. Released whenever there is physical activity/when the body is working hard, in labour they will help reduce pain and help the woman feel calm and 'zoned out'. Interruptions and chatter take you out of this zone, so keep this to a minimum to allow yourself to get into a rhythm. This is where your birth partner can really help in protecting your environment.

What will help you feel safe, secure and uninhibited?

- Lights out / lights low. This is the big one. Melatonin is a hormone that helps us sleep and its production peaks when it is dark. Melatonin helps with the release of oxytocin so keeping things dimly lit will help with this process. If you are planning a homebirth you will have more control over lighting, but you can still achieve this on the birth centre or labour ward as they both usually have dimmer switches. You could if you wanted to bring in portable blackout blinds, battery-operated candles or fairy lights for gentle, soft lighting, or bring in an eye mask or even sunglasses to shut out the outside world. The room is yours to make your own.

- Touch (if wanted!) – hugging, kissing, cuddling, stroking/massage – loving touch helps to release oxytocin and endorphins. A long hug from your partner or birth partner will make you feel safe; his or her familiar scent will settle and calm you.

45

- Movement – try rocking, swaying, using a birth ball, using the lowered bed as a prop to lean on rather than lay on, making a figure of 8 with your hips, getting on all-fours and leaning back and forth, sitting on the toilet: follow your body's lead. Movement helps the baby get into a good position and makes things feel more manageable for the mother.

- Quiet. This is not saying you cannot interact with or talk to anyone, but keeping interruptions to a minimum, and avoiding complex questions that take you out of your zone and stimulate your neocortex, is key. Birth can of course be noisy, and making sounds can be releasing. But make sure the environment you are in lends itself to letting you release, relax and go into yourself. Think of our mammal friends again and how and where they give birth. Each interrupted surge is one that is less efficient. Make each incredible, amazing and powerful surge count.

- Senses. Smell is one of the most powerful. The familiar smell of home, whether on a blanket, pillow or pyjamas, or a scent that you like on to a piece of fabric, such as a few drops of lavender oil, can increase comfort levels. If you've practiced using hypnobirthing use the same scent you used when doing your practice.

Sounds – play one of the MP3s included with this book that you have been listening to, its familiarity and the calming background music will ground you. You can also get a music play list together, or bring in ear plugs to block out the outside world.

- Letting go of fears and trusting your body knows how to birth your baby. There are practical tools on how to start working on this later in the book.

- Birth partners. Your input is so important! Ensure the birth plan is read (we all know birth preferences need to be flexible, but they are your hopes and wishes and it is important that they are read). Ensure your partner has access to food and drink. Control the environment; keep chatter at bay and protect your partner's space. Know that moments of self doubt are usual for a woman in labour and speak to the midwife out of earshot if you feel concerned by this. If you're unsure what to do, just think 'Am I/is this helping to make her feel safe, secure and private?'

When a woman has an undisturbed birth, her hormones flow perfectly, enhancing the safety of her and her baby. Interference with this hormonal flow can make birth more difficult and painful.

To conclude – of course, there is a lot we cannot control during birth. However, there is also a lot we can do to help ensure that it unfolds as comfortably and easily as possible.

Further reading

Lothian, Judith A. 'Do Not Disturb: The importance of privacy in labour' *Journal of Perinatal Education*, 2014.
http://www.ncbi.nlm.nih.gov. (Accessed August 2016)

Buckley, Sarah 'Undisturbed Birth', *AIMS Journal*, Vol 23, No.4, 2011.
www.aims.org.uk/Journal/Vol23No4/undisturbedBirth.htm

Barbeau, Beth 'Safer Birth in a Barn', *Midwifery Today*, 2007.
www.midwiferytoday.com (Accessed August 2016)

Buckley, Sarah 'Pain in Labour: Your hormones are your helpers', 2005 www.sarahbuckley.com/pain-in-labour-your-hormones-are-your-helpers-2 (accessed September 2016)

5

HOSPITAL BAG – WHAT TO PACK?

Some people like to pack two bags, one for labour and one for after the birth. It is a good idea for your birth partner to have their own bag too with a change of clothes, toiletries and snacks in (so they're not taking your stash!). If you are driving to the hospital or birth centre you could then leave the postnatal bag in the boot of the car, to save room.

A good tip is to lay out everything for your labour and birth bag on the bed and ask your partner to pack it. That way he or she will know exactly where everything is.

You will probably only use a few things that you bring, but as it can be hard to know what those things will be, packing for most eventualities is normal! Pack enough for one night. If you need more, your partner or a friend can go home and get things for you.

Here are some suggestions to consider:

- Your maternity notes if they are still the hand-held version.

- Several copies of your birth preferences sheet – you can stick one up on the wall too (bring sticky tack if you want to do this).

- A TENS machine with spare batteries and spare pads.

- Food – a selection of sweet and savoury items for you and your birth partner. You never know what you might fancy. If you like bananas, these provide good energy, as would dried fruits. Food for after the birth is good too, just in case it's the middle of the night and nothing is open.

- Sports cap water bottles or bendy straws so you can easily stay hydrated whatever position you are in.

- Phone charger – if you use your phone as your camera this is especially important for those first pictures! Likewise if you use your mobile phone to listen to hypnobirthing downloads.

- Phone numbers written down, in case the phone runs out and you are unable to charge it.

- Camera if you're not planning on using your phone.

- Toiletries.

- Ear plugs.

- A plain carrier oil or pregnancy massage oil for massages or putting a few drops of whatever smell you like (providing it is safe to inhale or have on your skin during labour) onto some fabric to aid relaxation. This is useful as if you get fed up with the aroma you can just remove the fabric.

- Music to listen to, or if hypnobirthing, the relaxation MP3s if they are not already downloaded onto your mobile phone. If relevant, take a battery-operated machine (laptop or a way to play your MP3s or music playlist), in case you are unable to plug things in.

- Things to make the environment as dark as possible – eye mask? Blackout blinds? The room is yours to change as you wish!

- Water spray to keep cool.

- A fan.

- A loose, comfortable change of clothes for you.

- Buy some cheap flannels, soak them in water and freeze them separately in sandwich bags. You can then take them out and use them on the back of your neck to cool you down.

- A hot water bottle – some women find warmth comforting.

- Dressing gown.

- Slippers.

- Socks.

- Flip-flops for the shower (non-slip!).

- A nightdress or big t-shirt.

- Lip balm.

- Hair band. If you have long hair, you might want it tied up.

- Pillows in your own pillow cases — the familiar scent of home will be very comforting and far more comfortable than the starchy hospital ones. Use non-white cases so the staff know the pillows are yours from home.

- Wipes for a quick freshen-up.

- Toiletries for a longer freshen-up! Treat yourself to a luxurious soap or shower gel. Just brushing your teeth can help to refresh you.

- A towel.

Postnatal bag

- Loose comfortable clothing for going home in.

- Nursing bra and breast pads.

- Maternity pads — you will likely need around 3-4 packets of these as they will require changing around every 2-3 hours for the first couple of days or so. Postnatal bleeding is normal and healthy after birth, whether caesarean or vaginal.

- Old or cheap, large and comfortable underwear.

- Hair brush.

- Pyjamas/something to relax in.

- Clothes for your baby such as a hat, a couple of all in one stretchy outfits, a cardigan, a couple of vests.

- A night shirt that opens at the front for easy skin to skin contact with your baby when feeding him.

- Baby blanket and/or snowsuit if the weather is cold.*

- Socks and or booties (depending on the weather).

- Nappies.

- Car seat in the car, already practised with or installed and ready to go!**

Remember to always remove bulky clothing before putting your baby into his or her car seat. If it is cold, you can tuck a blanket over the car seat straps once they are secured correctly.

**It is well worth getting your car seat checked to ensure that it is fitted correctly, as many are not and are therefore useless. There are independent car seat specialists, or sometimes local councils offer a free car sear checking service.*

I'M EXPECTING A BABY

6

THE BIRTH PARTNER'S ROLE

The role of the birth partner is so important. Sadly, it is not always possible to get continuous one-to-one support from our amazing but over-stretched midwives, so having the constant support of a familiar person is invaluable.

Birth partners can be the baby's father, dads, mums, partners, sisters, friends or a doula (more on doulas later). Usually a maximum of two supporters are allowed in the labour room or birth centre, although if you have a home birth you can have as many as you like.

Remember that the fewer interruptions the labouring woman has the better, and think about how you might feel giving birth in a room full of people, however lovely they are! Feeling observed can really hinder a labour, so it might be wise to keep birth partners to a minimum, though the choice is of course all yours.

Here are some tips for all you amazing birth partners out there:

Read up on labour and birth – starting with this guide. Knowledge is power and you need to be on board and stand the decisions and choices your partner will entially be making during labour and birth.

Attend as many classes as you can – NHS ones are free and they also often run breastfeeding workshops, which you can attend together. The National Childbirth Trust (NCT) offer paid for classes and some couples/women may be able to access classes at a subsidised cost. You can find out more on the website www.nct.org.uk.

Attending these classes will help you get a clearer idea of what the birth partner's role is, and the chance to discuss things with others is very helpful. NCT and any good hypnobirthing course go into this in detail and are well worth attending if you are able to.

Get practical and organised and think ahead in terms of how you will get to the hospital or birth centre. Will you drive? Take a cab? Or can a friend or family member be on call to transport you? If driving, have money ready for parking or set up a pay-as-you-go app on your phone to pay for parking. These can be quite handy, as you never know how long you will need and the apps usually send you a text to let you know your time is running out on the meter and you can top it up using your mobile phone. There are also websites where you can organise hiring a person's unused driveway which is situated close to the hospital – this is often cheaper than paying for meters. Ring around a few cab companies as not all will take a woman in labour.

Pack the hospital bag together so you both know where and what everything is.

Draw up a birth plan together. While it is valuable to plan, visualise and affirm your ideal birth, planning for all eventualities is useful as birth can be unpredictable at times. Once you have jotted down your wishes for all eventualities, such as if your partner is having her labour induced, put these 'what ifs' to one side and both go all out on focusing and visualising the birth you both want.

There is a birth preferences template in this book, or you can follow the NHS one or a template your midwife may give you.

Massage – the power of loving touch can be comforting and helps to produce the hormone oxytocin. It's a lovely way of saying you are there for her without needing to speak. This can be stroking, cuddling, kissing, hugging, holding – or none of these, as some women do not want to be touched during labour.

Practising massage techniques regularly in the weeks before labour starts is important, as your partner should not be negotiating on the day about the speed (ideally slow and rhythmic) and intensity of how she wants the massage to be. You can read more on massage later in the book.

Words of encouragement – if you choose to use the hypnobirthing relaxation scripts and MP3 downloads included in this book you can use these in labour if wanted.

It is usual for a woman to have moments of self doubt where she feels she cannot cope - gentle, calm, soothing words of encouragement may be helpful. Tell her how well she is doing, that she is birthing perfectly and beautifully and that it won't be long until you both meet your baby. Tell her how calm and strong she is. Keeping chat to a minimum is ideal and not chatting during the contraction to allow her to focus on it.

Positions – being gently active and encouraging your partner to get into upright, forward, open (think UFO!) positions can create almost a third more room for the baby to use – that is a considerable amount! Being 'UFO' means positions where she is sitting/standing and leaning forwards with legs open, or straddling a chair or the toilet seat backwards, or kneeling on the bed leaning over on a bean bag or cushions, etc.

If she is flat on her back this can hinder labour, as the sacrum at the lower back is not free to move back and create more space. On her back she isn't utilising the powerful force of gravity to help her and may feel less actively involved in the birth.

Lower or raise the bed when you arrive in the labour room, as she will then be less tempted to lay down on it (moving a labouring woman is not easy once she is settled on the bed!). She can then use the bed as a prop to lean on rather than lying on it. If she is tired, then laying on the bed on her side rather than her back is a good option.

Encourage her to circle on a birth ball the right size for her (her knees should be a little lower than her hips). Kneeling, squatting and all fours positions are great for labouring.

Breathing – remind your partner to breathe slowly and deeply, with the 'out' breath as long as, or if possible longer than, the 'in' breath. This provides oxygen to the baby and the mother's uterus.

Do your breathing practice together so you are familiar with how her relaxed breathing looks. If you notice she is starting to fall away from this, by panic breathing or holding her breath, co-breathe with her. Co-breathing is when you gently hold her or place your hands on her shoulders, and exaggeratedly breathe slowly and calmly in.... and out.... so she can mimic you and get back to her calm space and rhythm.

You can read more about breathing techniques, mantras, affirmations and ideas for visualisations later on in this book.

Think practically – keep an eye on your partner and her surrounding area. Could she do with another pillow? Is she well supported and comfortable with relaxed shoulders, or is she tense and could do with a massage or a hug? Is she having regular sips of water? Pass her the water bottle to encourage this.

Encourage her to empty her bladder every couple of hours as a full bladder can slow labour down.

Be her advocate. Take all questions in the first instance. This does not mean she cannot speak or engage with people, but when in active labour, particularly during a surge, she will need to stay focused and in her 'zone'. An interrupted surge is one that is less efficient. If you have something you are concerned about, quietly talk to the midwife about it out of her earshot, or at least wait until the contraction has passed.

Control the environment. You can read about hormones and environment in this book. Get the lights as low as possible, and use portable blackout blinds if needed. Keep interruptions to a minimum. Organise the music if this is what she wants. What scents does she like? Lavender is soothing and calming; she may like to breathe in some lavender essential oil or lavender spray on a pillow or piece of fabric. If doing hypnobirthing, what scent have you been using during your practice? Use this.

Switch your phone off – you need to be focusing only on her. Perhaps you could set up a Whatsapp group on your phone in advance for family and friends and let them know you will update them via this as and when there is any news.

If you are getting yourself a drink or a tea from the machine, offer your midwife one too. Chances are she has not had the time to have a break and would welcome a hot drink.

Handling questions and asking for information

Sometimes decisions need to be made in terms of your partner's labour/progress, or in advance of labour starting. Unless it is a clear emergency, always take the time to ask for more information. Your partner will need to consent to any procedure or next steps, but you can help her get the information she needs to make that decision. Read the chapter on Decision Making.

The questions below may be useful to ask if something is being suggested that you may not want:

- Thank you. I would very grateful to read up on the evidence on 'XYZ' – please can you point me to this to help us make our decision?

- Is this an emergency or is my partner/wife/baby in danger? If not, we'd like to wait a little longer to see how things progress and reassess in a little while.

- How will what you are suggesting affect the labour/birth/our baby?

- What other options are there?

- Please can you explain that to me in a bit more detail?

Think **BRAIN**: ask what are the:

Benefits   (of what is being offered)

Risks   (of what is being offered)

Alternatives   (to what is being offered)

Intuition   (what is your intuition saying/what is your 'gut' feeling?)

Nothing   (is there time to do nothing for a moment / think it over a little or talk it through, perhaps with a consultant midwife or senior midwife?)

BRAIN is a useful tool for many situations, such as if your partner is being offered any intervention, like having her waters broken or induction of labour.

Being a birth partner can be hard work! Take care of yourself too by staying hydrated and eating.

Feeling concerned about being a continual support to your partner? Are you very anxious? Anxiety and stress means you will be pumping adrenalin into her zone and she should not be concerning herself with how you are doing. If you feel this way, consider a second birth partner, someone who your partner feels safe and secure with and who will be a calming presence so you can duck out if things feel too much. You could consider hiring a doula.

A birth partner's to-do list for labour

There are many things that you can do to get your partner into a relaxed state. If you are opting to do the hypnobirthing/mindset elements which feature later in this book you will find a break down there with suggestions on what to do and when. In early labour remember there is usually plenty of time. You can:

- Snuggle up and put on a funny DVD/comedy to watch in early labour – cuddles, laughter and relaxation produces endorphins and makes us feel relaxed.

- Come up with other distractions for early labour – cook a nice meal together, play a board game, do crosswords, take a gentle local walk, etc.

- Make sure she is gently active, but also resting and conserving her energy.

- Have a carb-heavy meal, but nothing too rich or creamy as this may make her feel nauseous and her digestive system needs to rest ideally.

- Play gentle music, or listen to the hypnobirthing MP3/s.

- Encourage her to stay hydrated with sips of water.

- Run her a nice warm, candlelit bath.

- Have whichever essential oil blend she likes available for her to breathe in.

- Massage or hold her – touch releases endorphins and oxytocin.

- When you arrive in hospital be well versed in the birth plan and make sure the midwife reads it.

- Ask to change midwife if in the unlikely event you feel the birth plan is not being taken seriously or you do not feel supported. If this makes you feel awkward just remember this day is a shift in a midwife's career - but this is the only chance you will get to experience your baby's birth and having someone who is not supportive of your wishes is not acceptable.

- Be aware of your partner's health history so you can answer any questions if she wants this.

- When you arrive in your room, make it as dark as possible. Turn lights off and put blackout blinds up if you have them (you can get portable/travel ones to stick on windows).

- Remind her to empty her bladder every few hours as a full bladder can slow things down.

- Offer gentle, encouraging words, letting her know how amazingly well she is doing. Hearing your calm voice will help her feel supported.

A birth partner's to-do list for the third stage (delivery of the placenta)

- Keep her warm and relaxed. She may be shaky with adrenalin after the birth, which can delay the delivery of the placenta. Wrap a blanket around her.

- Encourage an all-fours or upright position.

- Suggest she empties her bladder if the placenta is slow in coming.

- Keep the lights low to maximise the hormone oxytocin, which is still needed.

- Make sure she has skin-to-skin with the baby, undisturbed, for at least an hour. If planning on breastfeeding, she can do this as this will produce a big hit of oxytocin, again helping to complete this last part of labour smoothly.

7

DOULAS – WHAT ARE THE BENEFITS?

What is a doula?

A doula is a non-medical birth professional that provides continuous, non-judgemental support for you and your birth partner. She is someone you would have interviewed in advance and spent some time with beforehand so you know you 'click' and feel comfortable with each other.

Her role is to never leave your side, to help your birth partner, and to advocate for you along with your partner, but not to make decisions for you or sway your decisions in any way. She will not take over your partner's important role.

She will be knowledgeable about birth and the hospital where you are birthing, but usually she is not medically trained (though some doulas may be midwives or have had medical training).

What are the benefits of a hiring a doula?

- She will be a constant presence — there is lots of evidence that when a woman has a constant, familiar presence during her birth, labour progresses better and she has less intervention.

- She will support you whatever your choices and wherever you choose to have your baby.

- Women who have continuous support are more likely to have spontaneous vaginal deliveries and report being more satisfied with their birth experience.

- Women who hire a doula are statistically more likely to feel less pain when a doula is present, so you are less likely to request pain relief such as an epidural.

- Continuous support means a woman is less likely to have an assisted birth and less likely to have a caesarean birth.

- Labour may be a bit shorter.

- She can, along with your partner, communicate to your care providers during labour, allowing you to keep your focus within.

- She can explain what is going on to you or your partner if you are unsure about things.

- She can provide physical support, along with your partner, such as massage, or helping you with movement and positions.

- If your partner is very anxious, she can take the pressure off him or her, reducing the adrenalin in the room and leaving you free to concentrate without worrying about your partner's needs or fears.

- If you choose, you can hire her postnatally too, to help with breastfeeding, taking the baby while you have a shower and possibly carrying out light household duties or preparing meals.

What won't a doula do?

- She will not undertake any medical tasks such as examinations or helping you to birth your baby.

- She will not give you medical advice or attempt to sway your decision-making.

- She won't change shifts like a midwife may during your birth.

Of course, hiring a doula costs money, and depending on where you are in the UK or the world prices can vary significantly. In the UK some doulas-in-training offer packages which are less expensive while they train.

Some women may be able to access support with funding, there are various projects available and you can find out if you could be eligible by visiting the website doula.org.uk or calling them for more information.

Further reading

Hodnett et al 'Continuous support for women during childbirth', NCBI. 2012. http://www.ncbi.nlm.nih.gov/pubmed/23076901 (Accessed August 2016)

Evidence Based Birth. 'The Evidence for Doulas'. Available at http://evidencebasedbirth.com/the-evidence-for-doulas/ (Accessed August 2016)

Quigley, C., Taut, C., Zigman, T. et al 'Association between home birth and breast feeding outcomes: a cross-sectional study in 28125 mother–infant pairs from Ireland and the UK', *BMJ* Open 2016. doi:10.1136/bmjopen-2015-010551 (Accessed via www.sarawickham.com/research-updates/home-birth-is-significantly-associated-with-breastfeeding/)

www.doula.org.uk/what-doulas-do/

8

INDEPENDENT MIDWIVES

Independent midwives are fully qualified, self-employed midwives. They carry out the same checks and assessments as their NHS colleagues, but rather than caring for many women, they care for the same woman throughout her pregnancy, being on call 24/7. They can also provide postnatal care if required, or include this in their package of care. Appointments will be flexible and longer so a woman and her partner have plenty of time to talk through any questions they have.

Research demonstrates many benefits of one-to-one care (called 'caseloading' in the NHS) but this care is not available in all areas of the UK. The benefits are:

- women are more likely to go into labour spontaneously.

- women are less likely to have an elective caesarean birth.

- women require fewer pain-relief drugs.

- breastfeeding rates improve.

Although there are no guarantees in life, including birth, choosing an independent midwife increases a woman's chances of having a straightforward birth because independent midwives provide continuity of care.

Most independent midwives attend homebirths, but they can also attend planned hospital births if they have a honourary contract with that hospital (if not they will attend as a birth partner). If you need to transfer in from home to hospital your midwife will go with you, but usually her NHS colleagues will take over your care and she can only stay in the capacity of a birth partner or advocate.

Like all midwives, independent midwives are regulated by the Nursing and Midwifery Council. However, they have more freedom to provide individualised care as they are less restricted by NHS guidelines and protocols.

There is of course a charge for their services, but you will likely be able to pay in instalments.

If you choose to book an independent midwife, this does not mean you cannot access NHS care. If you wish you can combine the two and accept the blood tests, scans and any emergency care required that the NHS provides.

There has been an issue with independent midwives' insurance meaning there was a halt to this valuable service. On 27 April, 2018 they state on their website imuk.org.uk that there are now some forms of insurance available to independent midwives meaning some can support women and families through birth. They recommend chatting to your local independent midwife to find out their position as the cost of the current insurance is such that it is not affordable to all and therefore a significant amount of midwives cannot work currently.

Further reading

http://www.imuk.org.uk/

https://www.nct.org.uk/pregnancy/choosing-independent-midwife

https://www.rcm.org.uk/news-views-and-analysis/news/one-to-one-care-backed-by-study

9

PLACE OF BIRTH – DECIDING WHERE TO HAVE YOUR BABY

At some point fairly early on in your pregnancy your midwife should talk to you about your options about where you would like to give birth to your baby. If this has not happened, you can request to go through it at your next appointment.

You can give birth at home, or in a midwife-led unit (otherwise known as a 'birth centre', or 'home from home') or in the main delivery unit (labour ward). Midwife-led units may be either freestanding (not attached to a hospital – though this is unlikely in the UK) or alongside (in the same building as the main labour ward – more usual).

It is well worth doing some research around each of the options discussed below. After all, when you plan a holiday chances are you spend at least a little (probably a lot!) of time researching your accommodation, or the resort.

Or, if you were planning a wedding, you would likely spend a fair amount of time planning and looking into the venue and making sure it suited your needs.

So take the time to research one of the biggest things you will ever do – have a baby.

You can compare different maternity statistics unit by unit by visiting http://www.which.co.uk/birth-choice

If you don't know your options you don't have any.

Home birth

Some women like the idea of giving birth at home – a place where they are in control and feel less like a patient, are able to have a bath, and to eat and drink whatever and whenever they want. It is easier to distract yourself at home and carry on as normal for longer. You can book a home birth with your midwife. When you go into labour you call your midwife and she or a member of her team, who you likely will already know or have met, will come out to you at home. When the birth is imminent, she will usually call a second midwife to help her. If you book a home birth you can change your mind at any time during your pregnancy, even during labour and instead opt to go to the birth centre or labour ward.

What are the benefits of a home birth?

- If you plan a home birth you are more likely to in advance have met the midwife who will take care of you during your labour (if your homebirth team offer what is called 'case loading' - where a named midwife will provide continuity of care). This can help you feel more comfortable and relaxed. Research has shown that labour usually progresses well at home when a woman knows her midwife.

- You are in your own domain, free to move as you wish and eat and drink whatever you fancy, whenever you fancy.

- If you need to transfer into hospital, your midwife will go with you. She may stay, or she may hand you over to the care of the hospital midwives on duty.

- There is less pressure to labour within a particular time-frame, which means that fewer interventions are offered to speed up your labour.

- Should you require medical intervention your midwife will arrange for you to go to your local hospital.

- There is less risk of infection at a home birth.

- You really do get one-to-one care, as the midwife will be focusing on you and your baby, no one else. She will be regularly listening in to your baby's heartbeat and will not hesitate to suggest you transfer in if she suspects there is a problem – something she will do long before any situation becomes an emergency.

- Home birth is strongly associated with improved breastfeeding outcomes.

- Midwives are highly skilled and trained to deal with emergencies.

The Birthplace study says for healthy women with a straightforward pregnancy that are having a second or subsequent baby, home births are safe for the baby and offer benefits for the mother and may offer the following benefits:

- a lower risk of having a caesarean section

- a lower risk of an assisted delivery, i.e. forceps or ventouse

- post-partum haemorrhage (excessive blood loss after having your baby) is significantly less likely after a home birth than after a hospital birth.

Home birth and safety

Medical emergencies can occur anywhere, regardless of where a woman gives birth – but do remember that giving birth is generally very safe.

Midwives are highly skilled and trained to deal with any urgent situations whilst calling for further help. For example, if a post-partum haemorrhage were to happen, the midwife would have the initial drugs necessary to manage this and would arrange prompt transfer into hospital.

In some cases women requesting a home birth may be encouraged to give birth in hospital, for example in the event of a pregnancy lasting longer than 42 weeks, or the baby being in a breech position. Some women with less straightforward pregnancies or less usual factors to consider choose to research the pros and cons of their specific situation and make an informed decision to still give birth at home.

What's available at a home birth?

- You can have a water birth at home if you hire a pool. Sometimes you can find second-hand ones online, and just buy a new liner. Your home birth team may have a pool you can hire.

- You can hire or buy a TENS machine and use this.

- You will have access to gas and air.

- You may have access to either pethidine or diamorphine (opiods).

NICE guidance states that you should be supported and informed about your birth place options. Your GP or midwife should not try to dissuade you from your choice unless they feel there is a genuine medical reason. If there is medical reason as to why something is being suggested then of course you'd be wise to discuss this and ask for sources of research and information on it. But the decision is always yours and you are free to make your own choices even if your caregivers do not agree with you.

Birth centre

Sometimes a birth centre is referred to as 'home from home' or 'midwife led suite'. Giving birth in a birth centre can be a great option for many women who have had straightforward pregnancies. Birth centres are run by midwives and do not routinely use medical interventions if labour progresses well. As many labours progress well, birth centres are a good alternative to giving birth in hospital.

Should a woman require any medical intervention she can transfer to the labour ward. Most birth centres are in the same building, even the same floor, as the main hospital/labour ward, which many women find reassuring.

Pros of using a birth centre

- Birth centres feel more homely and less clinical, which in turn can make you feel more relaxed.

- They are often more spacious, with more equipment available, such as birthing stools, birth balls and padded floors to comfortably kneel on.

- They may have a double bed available for after the birth for your birth partner to stay overnight, but this is sometimes tucked out of the way or folded up against the wall to encourage women not to hop up on it! This is because research shows that being upright and mobile during active labour has many benefits, shortening labour and making it feel more manageable.

- Within birth centres birth is seen as a normal event rather than a risky one, and having a straightforward birth is much more likely. Straightforward birth means giving birth vaginally, without any procedures or interventions such as assisted birth (forceps or ventouse), induction of labour or caesarean birth.

- Some centres allow you to stay in the room, with your partner and baby, for your whole stay, though you will need to transfer out if someone wants to use the room. Others request that you transfer to the postnatal ward at some point after the birth.

- The midwives who work in a birth centre have often chosen this environment as they have a passionate interest in supporting women to birth with little or no intervention.

Cons of using a birth centre

- If you decide you want an epidural you need to transfer to the labour ward. If your birth centre is not located within the hospital, ask your midwife which unit you would transfer to and how long this would take.

What's available at a birth centre?

- Very often pools are plumbed in or inflatable ones are available.

- You can hire or buy a TENS machine and use this.

- You will have access to entonox (gas and air).

- Sometimes the midwives are trained in and can offer aromatherapy massage or reflexology.

- Often you will be able to have pethidine or diamorphine for pain relief during labour should you want this.

- There is less equipment visible, which helps to give a feel of birth being a normal event.

- If your baby needed special care they would be transferred to the special care baby unit, which in most cases will be in the same building.

- While the transfer may not happen instantly unless it is an emergency, you can always change your mind and transfer out of the birth centre and onto the labour ward should you wish to – for example if you decided you now wanted an epidural (epidurals are not available on the birth centre).

Hospital birth/labour ward

Some women choose to give birth on the labour ward as they find it reassuring.

If a woman is having consultant led care she may be more likely to be offered the labour ward rather than the birth centre.

However, being in the hospital environment makes it more likely that you will be offered interventions, which is something to bear in mind. There is also less privacy in a hospital setting.

If you have had a complicated pregnancy or are likely to require a caesarean birth for medical reasons, you will be encouraged to give birth in hospital, on the labour ward.

Your care will still be provided by midwives, but doctors will be available if required. It is unlikely that you will have met your midwife in advance of your birth.

What is available on the labour ward?

- You will have access to an epidural, pethidine/diamorphine and entonox (gas and air).

- Some labour wards have birthing pools available – ask your midwife or check the Which? Birth website to see if bringing your own pool in is an option.

- Access to a special care baby unit.

Some women like to start in the birth centre and transfer to the labour ward if they feel they would like an epidural. Once you are in your room on the labour ward you can make it your own. You may like to:

- Dim the lights as low as you can.

- Cover windows with blackout blinds.

- Bring battery-operated fairy lights for a beautiful, soft glow.

- Cover any unused equipment with a scarf or blanket/towel to make it feel less clinical.

- Birth balls should be provided but you can bring your own.

- Raise or lower the bed so you are not tempted to get on it and not move around much thereafter.

- Bring music.

- Bring an essential oil of your choice to breathe in from a piece of fabric.

- Cover the clock so you are not focused on it.

Summary

It is your choice where you give birth. Take time to research all the options and choose wherever you think you will feel most relaxed.

You can always change your mind at any point, but if a home birth is something you are interested in you should make sure your midwives know this.

If you feel you are not being supported in your choices by your midwife or consultant you can contact a senior midwife, Consultant Midwife or Professional Maternity Advocate (PMA) by ringing your hospital or writing to/emailing him/her.

Further reading

Birthplace in England Research Programme, July 2016, NPEU. Available at https://www.npeu.ox.ac.uk/birthplace. (Accessed August 2016)

NCT. Birthplace Study. www.nct.org.uk (Accessed August 2016)
https://www.nct.org.uk/professional/research/pregnancy-birth-and-postnatal-care/birth/birthplace-study

http://www.which.co.uk/birth-choice/

I'M EXPECTING A BABY

10

POSITIONS FOR LABOUR

Before we get into the benefits of being upright and active for labour and birth, I'd like to mention optimal fetal positioning (OFP). This is when a woman uses her position and how she sits when pregnant to possibly help encourage the baby into a position where the back of their head is at the front, facing forward, rather than posterior or 'back to back' (meaning the baby's head and back is facing the mother's back).

A posterior position isn't a wrong or bad position. Perhaps the shape of your pelvis means that this is the position your baby chooses.

Quite often if a baby's position is posterior, or back to back, this can mean the mother has several days of on-off labour, making her overall labour slower. She often experiences back discomfort in between contractions meaning she cannot rest in between them which is tiring. The baby will then need to turn to be born which sometimes can take a long time. They don't always manage to do this and may need a little help out via an assisted birth.

There is not currently any robust evidence that being mindful of our position when pregnant encourages a baby into a certain position. However some healthcare professionals suggest the following ideas when going about your day as a way to attempt to encourage your baby into a head down position, with his back to your front or left side before labour starts.

You may also find that some of these positions and ideas help with back discomfort in the latter stages of pregnancy as well as during labour.

If this is something you'd like to look into you could try the following:

- Being more active assuming it's safe for you to do this. For example, try getting off the bus one stop earlier, swimming, pregnancy yoga, walking.
- Avoiding positions where you slouch, like sitting on a super soft chair or sofa that means you're leaning backwards. The baby's head is the heaviest part of the body meaning gravity could encourage this part to go towards her back – the lowest point.
- Instead try sitting on a dining room chair which is faced backwards, or sit on a birth ball to watch T.V. Some women bring birth balls into their work place to sit on and find that this helps to relieve back pain. The position you're in should be having your knees slightly lower than your hips so that your pelvis is slightly tipped forwards.
- Adopt an all fours position for a few minutes a day. This is also a good position to relief back pain when in labour.

Positions for labour and birth

Many people in the Western world, when asked to visualise a birth, will conjure up images of a woman flat on her back for both labour and birth. This is usually how birth is depicted on TV, in films and pretty much everywhere!

In hospitals the bed usually takes centre stage, and when the woman gets on it she goes from being active to being still, a passive patient. Some midwives may prefer a woman to be on the bed, and sometimes women may think they are expected to be on it. It is always your choice where and how you labour and give birth and you should be free to get into whatever position that you want to.

Being flat on your back and immobile during labour can make your contractions feel much more intense. You may also feel helpless and as if labour is happening to you, rather than you being actively involved in it. When you lie flat on your back the vessel which carries blood into your heart is restricted due to the weight of the uterus restricting the blood flow. Reduced blood and oxygen supply can lead to your baby becoming distressed, requiring intervention. If you are tired, side lying can be beneficial.

You could consider asking your birth partner to raise the bed when you get into your room so you can lean and use it as a prop, rather than being tempted to lie back on it. Or you can kneel on the bed itself over a pile of cushions or a bean bag.

The images overleaf show how a woman's position can restrict or create space within the pelvic cavity.

The sacrum is a triangular bone in the lower back, at the bottom of the spine. It is slightly mobile and in the birth process it actually moves a little to allow the head past.

Being upright and off your back in labour can create up to one third more room in the pelvis!

In this squatting position you can see that the sacrum is free and able to move back to widen the pelvic outlet.

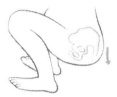

When a woman is in the semi sitting position, her body weight rests on her coccyx and the pelvic capacity is reduced.

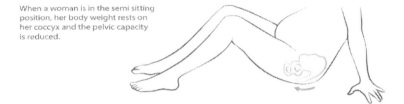

When a woman is in the reclining position the sacrum is immobile and the pelvic outlet narrows.

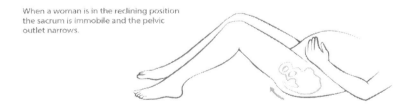

What are the benefits of upright positions in the first stage?

- More efficient surges.

- You feel more involved in your birth.

- The baby has a better oxygen supply.

- Movement is a good distraction for the mother.

- Birth partners can access your back or shoulders for massage.

- Squatting and all kneeling positions increase the diameter of the pelvic outlet.

- You make use of the powerful force of gravity

- Swaying, rocking or circling on a birth ball, walking and going up and down the stairs sideways or two at a time (assuming there is no pelvic girdle pain present) may help your baby get into a good position for birth.

- Upright positions in the first stage can mean a shorter first stage and less use of drugs and epidurals.

What are the benefits of upright positions in the second stage?

- A shorter second stage.

- Fewer instrumental births (use of forceps and ventouse) and fewer episiotomies (surgical cuts to the perineum).

- Your birth partner can easily give you massage and hugs.

- The use of a ball in second stage is thought to be supportive, providing counter pressure on the perineum and helping the baby descend during second stage pushing. It can also maximise pelvic capacity though of course you'll need to be off the ball to actually give birth.

Giving birth lying laterally (on your side) has been shown to have a protective effect on the perineum.

Below are some ideas for positions in labour/birth

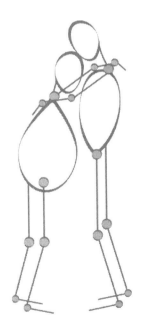

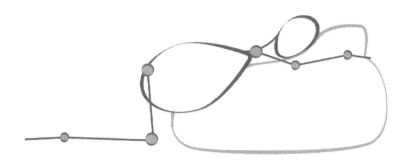

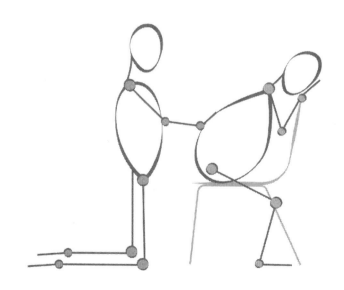

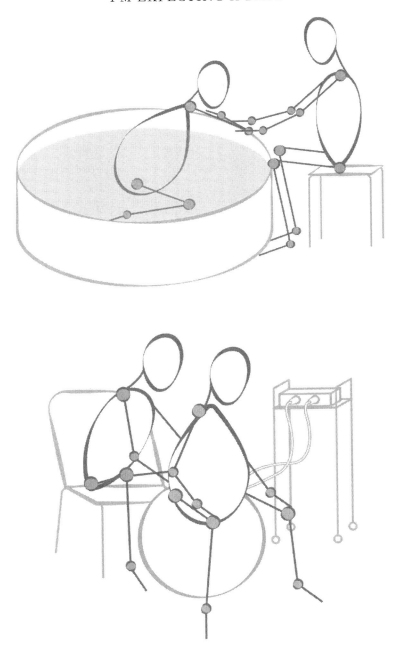

In the last picture the woman is being monitored electronically to keep a closer eye on her baby's wellbeing. If you need to have your labour more closely monitored you can request that this is all set up whilst you are on the birth ball. You will then be able to remain far more active than if it's all set up when you are laying on the bed. You should not have your movement restricted when you are in labour.

Further reading

'Evidence-based guidelines for midwifery-led care in labour. Positions for Labour and Birth', Royal College of Midwives https://www.rcm.org.uk/sites/default/files/Positions%20for%20Labour%20and%20Birth.pdf

11

BREATHING IN LABOUR

The Autonomic Nervous System (ANS) controls our body's involuntary functions like keeping our heart beating, controlling blood pressure and keeping us breathing all without us having to think about it. It is divided into two parts - the sympathetic part ('fight or flight') and the parasympathetic part ('rest and digest') which gets things back to normal after any danger has passed, calming and relaxing the body.

Slow, relaxed, rhythmic breathing activates the relaxation response of your parasympathetic nervous system – the 'rest and digest' response. It causes your nervous system to change its state into one of calm - calming both the body and the mind.

By the time you are ready to give birth your uterus will be the strongest, largest muscle in your body. To function well and efficiently, it needs a good blood and oxygen supply. Slow, calm breathing will help with this, keeping you focused and conserving energy.

Sometimes a woman in labour will tense her body and hold her breath during surges, which increases her adrenalin levels and reduces oxytocin. In turn, this soon starts to makes her feel panicky and she greets the next surge with fear and anxiety,

triggering the sympathetic part of the nervous
body assumes there is a threat to be managed so .
'fight or flight' response. Blood is diverted from the
this is not deemed a useful organ when faced with . unreat
(even though the threat is imagined, the mind does not know
this and will think 'now is not a time to be giving birth!') so
that blood flow to the arms, legs and brain can be increased to
work out and deal with whether to 'fight' or 'flight'.

Breathing becomes shallow, oxygen is decreased for you and
your baby and it isn't long until you feel light-headed and out
of control. This type of breathing cannot be sustained for long
and quickly exhausts you.

Now that the uterus doesn't have the tools of oxygen and a
good blood flow and it won't be long until the muscles gets
tired, causing unnecessary pain in labour and making surges
less efficient. Our hands and our jaw can clench and shoulders
tense up around our ears, making them feel tight.

The good news is there's a lot you can do to help to keep your
breathing calm and in control during the active stage of labour,
below are some tips:

- When you feel you no longer want to chat through
  your surges, this is the time to start your birth breathing
  – though of course you can start earlier if you wish to.

- Surges (contractions) are like waves. They start of mild,
  slowly building up until they reach a peak of intensity
  lasting around 20-30 seconds, and then peter off down
  the other side. There is then a gap where no sensation
  is felt until the next one begins.

- When you feel the contraction starting, a sighing out breath can shake off tension that has built up or crept into your body (see 'pre surge body scan in the hypnobirthing chapter). Quickly assess your posture — where are you tense? Make every muscle floppy and loose. Open your hands/palms, this signals relaxation.

- Closing your eyes can help take your focus within. Some women like to wear eye masks to help with this.

- Breathe deeply in through your nose (or mouth if you have a blocked nose) — focusing on filling your lungs to their capacity, breathing deep into your stomach, creating space for your baby in the uterus. When you have filled your lungs, slowly let the breath out through a soft, slightly open mouth, sighing out softly. Doing this means it takes longer for the out breath to complete than the in breath and this is important in keeping you calm. Sighing releases tension so try slowly sighing out the out breath to keep relaxed.

- Any visualisations around opening and softening may be a good focus seeing as this is what you want your body to do.

- Repeat these long, slow, deep breaths in, and out, until you feel the surge peter out and if you wish you can end the surge with a short sigh, releasing any last bit of tension.

- Focus on the present moment, not what's ahead. 'Right now I am breathing slowly and softly through this surge'.

- Visualisations, mantras and affirmations are powerful! For example 'Breathing in relaxation, breathing out softness/tension/stress. Tell your brain what you want your body to do clearly and simply. We go through this more later on.

- Try breathing in deeply and saying 'relax, relax, relax' to yourself on the out breath.

- Use visualisations such as imagining seeing your out breath slowly being released, using colour can help with this.

- Saying the word 'yes' is surprisingly freeing! 'No' is such a closed word, whereas mentally (or out loud!) saying 'yes, yes, yes' slowly and calmly is empowering.

- Try counted breathing – breathe in, 2, 3, 4, breathe out, 2..., 3..., 4..., 5..., 6..., 7..., 8... Pregnant women have reduced lung capacity, so do not feel disheartened if you cannot get much of a long out breath when practising before your baby arrives. You may find that after around 36 weeks, as the baby engages into your pelvis, that you have better lung capacity. Many women find with practice they're able to elongate their breath more, but don't force things so you feel uncomfortable. The breathing should feel pleasant and calming as you practice.

- Keep your jaw soft, teeth unclenched, shoulders relaxed.

tise breathing with your birth partner so they know you look and act when you are doing your relaxed breathing. They will then be able to recognise when you are not doing this in labour. If they notice you have started panic breathing, you can do co-breathing. As mentioned earlier, co-breathing is when your partner gently gets your attention by holding you or looking into your eyes and breathes slowly and deeply so you can mirror him or her and get your rhythm back.

Remember that in between surges nothing will be felt – use this time to have a sip of water, or a nibble of something to eat, or to use the bathroom.

Take one surge at a time, each one is bringing you one step closer to meeting your baby.

Try this practice contraction exercise with your birth partner or just yourself.

In active labour, surges usually last around 45-60 seconds so for the purpose of this exercise, let's use 50 seconds.

1. Get a stopwatch or timer – most mobile phones have one in the clock/alarm settings.

2. Sit with your birth partner and do nothing except count how many 'normal' breaths you do in a 50 second period. Breathing in then out is one breath. In and out again is two breaths, and so on.

3. Make a note of how many breaths you did in a 50 second period.

4. Reset the stopwatch.

5. Put on some gentle, soothing music.

6. Start the stopwatch.

7. This time imagine you can feel a surge building so you greet it with a sigh and do the pre-surge body scan.

8. Get into one of the birthing positions, rock and sway.

9. Take a long, deep, slow breath in, and if possible, release a longer out breath. Try counted breathing or a visualisation.

10. Have your partner massage you if they're around.

11. After 50 seconds is up note how many breaths you did.

Most people are surprised to note that second time around seems a lot faster! They usually report doing fewer breaths the second time, and find that after the pre-surge body scan it takes something between 3-5 lovely deep breaths rather than the usual 10–15 normal breaths.

This exercise is a great way for you both to see the benefits of distraction in the form of visualisation, counting, movement and music.

It's reassuring to know that in around 3-5 breaths your surge will be finished and it will have been beautifully efficient, with great blood flow and oxygen for you and your baby.

Remember that at the peak of the surge, where it is at its most powerful, is usually around 20-30 seconds which is pretty much 1-1.5 breaths in... and out.... You are now one big step closer to meeting your baby.

Breathing for the second stage (the pushing, nudging or breathing down stage)

When your cervix is fully dilated (and you do not have an epidural in place), at some point most women feel an irresistible urge to push or bear down. This is often a very instinctive stage of labour so just follow your body's lead: it knows what it's doing.

As you will feel a powerful urge to push during this stage, it is best to avoid 'coached pushing' as it really is not needed! Coached pushing involves sustained breath-holding and being directed when and how to push ('take a deep breath in, hold it, and push! Push! Push!'). This is not recommended unless there is a medical emergency, as it is disempowering and may cause harm. It is associated with raised blood pressure and reduced oxygen being sent to the baby, compromising the baby's oxygen supply, and there is some evidence to suggest it may weaken the pelvic floor. It is also exhausting, unpleasant, and may leave you feeling lightheaded. Instead, follow your body's lead.

You may like to take a deep breath in through your nose and let the breath out through your nose (or mouth if you prefer), firmly but not forcefully, still keeping the jaw loose. Focusing *downwards* towards your pelvic floor will help you to encourage your baby downwards. This type of breathing keeps you energised and maintains a good flow of oxygen. It can help to visualise how a coffee plunger gets pushed down and think of the out breath operating like this. You can visualise your out breath moving down the back of your throat towards your pelvic floor as a powerful but gentle force helping to nudge your baby on his journey into the world. It is more effective to get two or three short pushes/nudges in with each contraction rather than one long breath-holding push.

If you've had an epidural, your midwife will normally advise you to delay pushing for up to one or two hours from the time you are fully dilated before you start pushing, as this gives your baby a chance to descend further into your pelvis. As an epidural numbs a woman from the waist down, it can be hard to know when to push - work with your midwife to find out what breathing techniques may help at this time.

Most women make some noises when pushing/breathing down! Often it is instinctive and it's perfectly normal to make some noise during this expulsive stage of labour. Noise is freeing and helpful and should not be restricted in any way.

A breathing and positive affirmations MP3 is included as part of your MP3 downloads with this book.

Further reading

'Evidence Based Guidelines for Midwifery-Led Care in Labour. Second Stage of Labour', Royal College of Midwives, 2012. (Accessed   via https://www.rcm.org.uk/sites/default/files/Second%20Stage%20of%20Labour.pdf)

Heli, S, Confident Birth, Pinter & Martin

12

MASSAGE IN LABOUR

Receiving massage during labour can be comforting and bring you closer to your birth partner. It is a way of communicating without words and a way for your partner letting you know they are there for you. Massage also stimulates endorphin and oxytocin production. Some essential oils are safe to use, diluted in a carrier oil, and there's more on this later. However, some women prefer not to be touched during labour and that is fine too.

Practise the massage techniques during your pregnancy so that when you are in labour your partner knows what you like, what you don't like and how much pressure to use. Make sure that he or she is well versed in slow, rhythmic massage. You do not want to be negotiating this kind of thing on the day!

Any kind of touch can be comforting. Kissing, cuddling, hugging, holding and stroking are all great.

Massage of the back, shoulders, neck, legs and hands can feel good. Massage of the feet can feel pleasant too, even if this is not usually your thing. For feet the pressure should be firm or it will feel annoyingly tickly.

ught strokes are when your partner uses the backs of his or her fingers to gently stroke you. Some women like this, others do not. If it irritates you, you can ask your partner to use their flattened palms rather than fingertips to stroke more firmly.

When labour becomes more intense, some women like to have a counter-pressure back massage during a contraction. Partners can use their knuckles, thumbs, the heels of their hands or even tennis balls to massage the back area. When using firm pressure it is important to avoid the spine and instead focus on the fleshier parts, such as the tops and sides of the hips and buttocks, or circle around the sacrum.

If you prefer not to have your body touched, having your face or hair stroked may be soothing, or having your hands massaged.

Essential oils are powerful substances and can interfere with contractions if used incorrectly. Some suggestions for essential oils are: Lavender, Jasmine, Frankincense (great for anxiety), Camomile, Rose or a citrus oil. Clary Sage may encourage more contractions but can make some women feel very sick. If you want to use essential oils check with a qualified aromatherapist that the ones you plan to use are safe for labour. Always dilute essential oils with a carrier oil or base oil - 1 percent - 1 drop to 5ml of carrier oil. Perhaps consider not using oils on the front of the body as the strong smell may get in the way of the baby's ability to locate the breasts for feeding.

Below are some massage techniques to try.

Below are some ideas for massage during labour

Following 'A' is useful if a woman is using a TENS machine

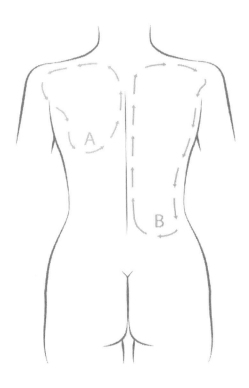

Massaging the sacrum firmly in a circular motion can feel great. You can use the heel of the hand, or even tennis balls — but these can give quite a strong pressure so be aware

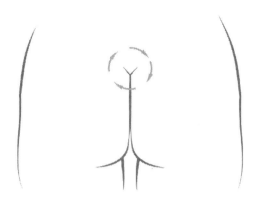

Sometimes it's not possible to get to the back, in which case a firm leg and/or foot massage is good

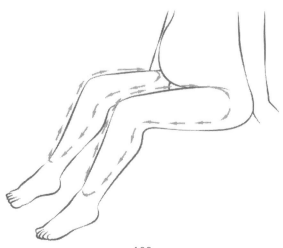

We can hold quite a bit of tension in our hands – and again, if the back cannot be accessed, a hand massage can be comforting. Below is a hand massage routine, but there are no real rules, so go with what you enjoy

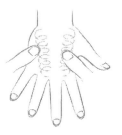 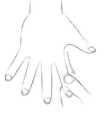

Further reading

Silva Gallo, R.B., Santana, L.S., Jorge-Ferreira, C.H., et al 'Massage reduced severity of pain during labour: a randomised trial', *J Physiother* 59(2):109-16, 2012.

13

PREPARING YOUR MIND FOR BIRTH

Giving birth is a huge physical feat, but your mind also has a huge role to play. The power of the mind is a vast subject, but in this chapter we look at the power of the mind for labour and birth. You will find more on this within the Hypnobirthing chapter.

When a woman finds out she is pregnant, she may start taking vitamins, pay attention to her diet and stop drinking alcohol, to keep her body and baby healthy. But how many women think about giving their mindset a makeover?

Birth is a normal, natural event. It is certainly challenging – but we are fortunate that in our culture it is no longer a life-threatening event, thanks to advances in hygiene and antenatal and postnatal care. However, I will take a bet that most women are absolutely terrified of giving birth – and it is no wonder, when you consider what we have been fed all our lives by media and well-meaning friends and family.

Think about it. Have you ever seen a positive birth on TV, or in a film? Have you heard many positive birth stories from friends or read any positive birth articles in magazines?

When you consider how birth is portrayed on TV, you probably think of something like this: a woman's waters break dramatically. She clutches her stomach in immediate agony. She is rushed to hospital, in great pain. She lies flat on her back in hospital, screaming, while she is shouted at to 'Push! Push! Push!'. She is surrounded by people and panic. The baby is 'delivered' by staff telling her what to do.

No wonder many women are anxious about birth!

The problem is that unless you have given birth positively before, these negative stories and images are the ones your mind will 'go to' when you are in labour, and this can dramatically affect how your body works. These negative images and birth stories chip away at a woman's confidence in her ability to birth her baby, taking away trust and faith in her perfectly designed, incredible body and replacing this with anxiety and fear. We go into this in more detail later, but it is explained a little below.

Many of you will have heard of the conscious and subconscious mind. The subconscious mind is like a library, or a memory bank, and its capacity is vast. It stores everything that has ever happened to you, and its purpose is to store and retrieve data and ensure you respond in the way in which you are 'programmed'.

If you have not given birth before, the subconscious mind will use whatever reference material it has. For the majority of women this will be what they have seen and heard about birth on TV and from friends and family. Usually, though of course not always, this section of their 'mind library' is full of negativity and fear. So when a woman goes into labour, the subconscious thinks 'birth is not safe, it hurts and it's frightening', which provokes fear and raises adrenalin levels setting off a chain reaction that can hinder and slow down labour.

The good news is there is a lot you can do to reboot and reprogramme the birth section of your mind library. You can:

- Stop watching programmes that depict birth negatively. They feed the subconscious with negative birth fodder that it will access and go to when it is your turn to give birth.

- Watch positive births on YouTube (to do the opposite of the above!) – there are tons out there.

- Look into mindset strategies such as hypnobirthing.

- Read positive birth stories on sites such as 'Tell me a good birth story'. You will find some positive hypnobirthing birth stories within the Hypnobirthing chapter, or sign up to hypnobirthing Facebook pages to have your news feed full of birth positivity.

- Find out about your local Positive Birth meet-up group http://www.positivebirthmovement.org/ and borrow or buy positive birth books. Web links and book suggestions can be found at the end of the book.

- Close your ears to negative birth stories – don't be afraid to stop someone in their tracks by saying 'I'd love to hear your birth story once I've had my baby' (unless it is super positive).

- Listen to the hypnobirthing MP3s included in this book. They are simply positive guided relaxations. You can fall asleep to them, or listen to the positive affirmations while you get ready for work, cook or potter about at home.

- Choose some affirmations that you like from this book, from Pinterest, or just make up your own. Stick at least one up where you will notice it each day. Say it out loud, say it in your head. If you think it's a load of rubbish then say it 10 times more!

- Use visualisation. All the top sports competitors use this tool. There is a ton of evidence around it working – see the section below.

- Breathing – practise your breathing techniques every day, at random moments such as on a busy train or bus, or when you are feeling wound up by a colleague – as well as with your partner and before you go to sleep or get out of bed in the morning.

- Positions for labour – reboot the mind so it knows you don't have to be on your back! Try out the positions included in this book. Practise them alone, with breathing, with your partner. If you practice them in advance you are more likely to use them on the day.

- Attend a good pregnancy yoga class from as early as possible as during these sessions you'll spend time practicing birth positions, breathing and enjoy guided relaxations.

- Knowledge – knowledge is power! After all, if you don't know your options, you don't have any. Understand how your amazing body works. Learn what helps and hinders labour. We cover all this in this book, but don't let that stop you from reading more and more.

Mind your language. Tune into how you speak to yourself. Are you talking positively to yourself about birth?

A woman in labour is an incredible and strong force! I am continually amazed at our power. Despite this, it doesn't take much to knock a woman's confidence when she is in the vulnerable state of giving birth – and many things can do this, words being one of them.

How information is relayed and the choice of words used can make a big difference. Couples who have prepared with hypnobirthing may choose to use the word 'surge' or 'wave' instead of the word 'contraction'. A surge of energy or a wave in the sea will have a rhythm to it, it begins, builds, peaks and then peters off. Just like a contraction, but a far nicer way of picturing and feeling it – and can also help with visualisations during labour. You know when it starts that it will build and after around a minute, will be gone.

You may also like to consider in advance not only how you feel about having internal examinations to establish (amongst other things) how dilated your cervix is, but how you'd like this information delivered to you.

For example, would you like your partner to relay this information to you, or are you happy for the midwife to tell you? Remember that an examination only offers a snap shot of time and it may have taken you 'X' amount of hours to get to being say 5cm dilated, but this doesn't mean that it will take the same time again to get further on.

Rather than being told the cold, hard facts of how many centimetres dilated you are perhaps you'd find it easier to stay in a relaxed and confident zone if you heard the information this way:

"You are progressing beautifully [insert how many c.m. if this is something you really want to know]! You have so much confidence and calmness about you. Just keep taking one surge at a time and know that each surge is bringing you closer to meeting your baby."

"Words are, of course, the most powerful drug used by mankind" – *Rudyard Kipling*

Of course, Kipling is describing how a certain choice of words can change and influence how a person thinks and feels.

How do you want to receive information when in labour?

The importance of visualisation and affirmations

According to research using brain imagery, visualisation works because neurons (which are cells that transmit information) in our brains interpret imagery as a real event. When we visualise an act, the brain generates an impulse that tells our neurons to 'perform' the act (the 'act' in our case being a positive and calm birth experience). It is like a mental warm-up, conditioning your mind to think clearly and recognise how it will act positively in response to certain events, situations or pressures.

Firing up our neurons with visualisation creates a new neural pathway which in turn works with our brain to create new learned behaviours, priming our body to act in a way consistent to that which we visualised. All of this occurs without actually experiencing the physical activity.

There are two types of visualisation – **outcome visualisation** where you would spend time visualising the end result - you both, relaxed and elated with your baby in your arms feeling amazing and proud!

The second type of visualization is **process visualisation**. This involves envisioning each of the actions necessary to achieve the outcome you want, for example, see you both regularly doing your hypnobirthing practice and feeling your confidence grow. Imagine yourself having a moment of self doubt during labour as it all intensifies - and visualise what you do to break through this, etc. (*Niles, Frank: Using Visualisation to Achieve your Goals*)

You can use the written word if preferred, or combine both this and mental imagery. You can also get really creative if this is your thing and create a birth vision board using pictures, quotes and affirmations. For both types of visualisation it's good to bring as much detail in as possible, using all of the senses.

So take time to regularly imagine how your birth will be. How smooth and calm it will be. Add as much detail as possible. This is a lovely thing to do before bed so that you fall asleep with your positive birth story in your head rather than a bad news story, or worrying about what you need to get done at work the next day.

Here are some suggestions you can use when using visualisation techniques for your baby's birth:

- Who will be there, picture them. What are they wearing, saying, doing.

- What will it smell like - is there a scent you like that you will be bringing with you? It's good to use the same scent that you used during your practice as this will act as a trigger, reminding of a time when you felt calm, confident and trusting of your body. Or perhaps a lavender pillow, or a pillow from your bed at home that smells of your familiar washing powder/home rather than a starchy hospital smell.

- What will the atmosphere be like? How dark, peaceful and soothing will it be? Perhaps you will have battery operated candles or fairy lights set up to create a spa-like zone.

- How will you feel when you are in labour? How relaxed, powerful and calm!

- What can you hear – particular music? Soothing words from your caregivers? One of the MP3s, or your partner's familiar voice?

- What can you feel – your partner massaging you or a lovely bear hug? Or no touch, but feeling your deep calming breaths in.... and out.... Can you feel the soft material of your favourite pyjamas or perhaps the warm water of the birthing pool...

- See yourself looking at your baby in your arms – you did it! How amazing and in awe will you feel? Feel the joy, the pride, the excitement. Feel your baby's warm, soft skin and her weight in your arms.

- Add in as much precise detail as is possible involving all of your senses.

Go and visit where you will be giving birth – look at the birth centre or the labour ward. If this is not possible, most maternity wards have online tours you can do. You need to be able to conjure up as many details as possible when visualising your birth positively.

Affirmations

The idea of affirmations – which are statements said or written down repeatedly with confidence - is that when we repeat something over and over, it convinces our mind that it is true.

Affirmations have the ability to program your mind into believing what it is you are repeatedly stating or writing down. This is because the mind doesn't know the difference between what is real or fantasy – like when you watch a sad film and start to cry or a comedy and start to laugh.

When you say or write your affirmations, do so in the present tense, as if they are happening now, not in the future. Some examples are given below, though you can of course create your own. Even if you only find one you like, focus on that.

Write or type it out and stick it up around your home on the wall, the fridge, even the back of the toilet door! Anywhere you will notice them on a daily basis. It's all about the repetition to embed the positivity firmly in your mind so you start to change the way you think and feel about birth, replacing fear with confidence and trust.

There are numerous birth affirmations out there and a quick look online will bring them up. You will find positive affirmations on the *Breathing & Positive Affirmations MP3* included with this book.

Below are some affirmation suggestions.

I give birth easily and calmly.

My birth is smooth and comfortable.

I believe I can and so I will.

Each breath and surge (or contraction) brings my baby closer to me.

Women all over the world are giving birth with me.

Breathing deeply and slowly relaxes my muscles, making my labour comfortable.

My body knows how to birth my baby.

I am strong and I trust my body knows what to do.

I relax into each surge, maximising oxygen to me and my baby.

I keep gently active, I create space for my baby to be born swiftly and easily.

All is well.

*Surges are powerful and strong, but they are not stronger then me because they **are** me.*

I am using my surges to birth my baby.

I relax and let my body take over to birth my baby.

I am ready and looking forward to the birth of my baby.

I breathe in relaxation, I breathe out softness.

As labour progresses my relaxation deepens.

Whatever turn my birth takes, I remain calm and in control.

I am able to make decisions about my birth clearly and calmly.

Don't worry if this feels 'fake', or you don't believe it. In fact if you feel sceptical, increase the amount of visualisation and affirmations you do each day.

Releasing Fears

As we've seen, how birth is depicted in our culture means that women are understandably fearful of it. What we focus on tends to become our reality, so spending time before your birth releasing your fears and turning them into positive feelings can be really powerful. This is a big part of hypnobirthing which you'll read about later.

You know from reading about some of the hormones in labour that fear can slow things down and make things feel more uncomfortable than they need to be. What we feel in our minds has a real impact on our bodies.

Have you ever had a job you disliked, and found yourself getting that 'Sunday blues' feeling, when your heart literally sank at the thought of going to work on Monday? Or have you ever remembered an embarrassing situation and found yourself cringing, as the feelings and physical sensations you felt at the time come flooding back to you? What about remembering a good night out with friends? Do you find yourself smiling or laughing to yourself when remembering the events of a fun evening?

These events aren't real right now – you're creating or recreating them in your mind – but your mind can't tell the difference between real and imagined events and reacts by bringing up the relevant emotions and physical sensations regardless.

The Fear-Pain-Tension cycle

In the 1930s, obstetrician Dr Grantly Dick-Read formulated what he called the Fear-Pain-Tension cycle. When we are fearful we become tense, and this tension causes pain. The pain then further fuels the fear, and so the cycle continues.

In preparation for labour and birth a woman's uterus has developed many more blood vessels than that of a non-pregnant woman as the increased circulation is necessary for efficient muscular action.

When we are tense and in pain we understandably feel panicky and this panicky feeling can tip us into 'freeze, fight or flight' mode. The fight or flight instinct comes from our old mammalian brain and is designed to keep us safe, so it overrides the logical part of our brain. This is what happens:

- Our breathing becomes shallow and rapid, heart rate increases

- We feel nauseous

- We may feel sweaty or have a dry mouth

- Blood is diverted away from non-essential organs to the legs, arms and brain so we are primed to either freeze (play dead), fight or run (flight).

- During birth, this means that the blood will be drained from the uterus, as it is not deemed an essential organ when the body is in fight or flight mode/an emergency situation.

- The uterus cannot work efficiently with a poor blood and oxygen supply.

- The result is that the birth process feels more painful and frightening.

Dick-Read believed that when fear is removed, tension is reduced, or even removed altogether, which means that the uterus is able to work to its full capacity as it is perfectly designed to do.

While giving birth is no walk in the park – after all, something utterly incredible is taking place – it does not need to be full of terror, tension and agonising pain. Spending time understanding how the body works in labour and what can hinder it helps a lot, and spending time releasing any fear you have around childbirth will be very beneficial too.

Releasing fear is important for birth partners too – if they can address their concerns about birth before the big day, they won't be bringing unwelcome anxiety, adrenalin and stress into the birth room.

Spend a little time thinking about your concerns around labour and birth.

- Do you have past experiences to call upon?

- What birth 'horror stories' have you heard that have particularly stuck in your mind? Remember – these are **not** your stories!

- Has a friend or family member had a difficult birth?

It may feel easier and more comfortable to ignore these concerns but acknowledging them will help you to release them. If you have a partner, talk through your fears together. If any fears are linked with a past birth, ask to go through your notes with a senior midwife to help you understand what happened and why. Try to release as much fear as much as you can before your birth.

Some things you may like to consider

- Are you happy with where you are planning on giving birth or would you like to change this?

- Can you remember details from a less than positive birth story which are sticking in your mind and making you worry?

- Do you feel concerned or overwhelmed about any particular issues?

- Are you worried about lack of support during or after the birth? If so, who else can you call on? Is a doula an option?

- Is your partner on board with your birth wishes? Again, if not, is a doula or additional birth partner an option?

Harbouring fear can hinder the smooth progress of your labour. Spending time releasing these concerns will help your baby and body now, and when you go into labour. It may be useful to see a qualified and experienced hypnotherapist if fear still feels very strong, or you have a difficult past birth experience to work through.

Once you have identified any fears you can try the following:

- Write them down. Read them out. Then tear them up into tiny pieces.

- Visualise putting all the fears into the basket of a hot air balloon. See yourself setting it free. Watch it float away until it is a tiny dot, then gone – taking its now vanished fears with it.

- As each fear comes up, see it as a cloud leaving your head, floating upwards, drifting away, until you can see it no more.

These are just a few ideas. You will find more on this later in the book.

Further reading

Mongan, Marie F. *Hypnobirthing*, third edition, Souvenir Press, 2008.

Dick-Read, Grantly *Childbirth Without Fear*, Pinter & Martin, 2004.

14

HYPNOBIRTHING

Some people may be put off by the word 'hypnobirthing'. If you know nothing about hypnobirthing, the word may conjure up images of stage hypnosis where people are hypnotised to eat onions as if they were apples, swirly patterns, mind control and goodness knows what else! This is thanks to stage hypnosis shown on some television programmes, which is done for entertainment purposes only.

We all enter the state of hypnosis several times a day, so it is a very familiar, natural state to our minds and bodies - we can all do it. Ever relaxed watching a film and become totally engrossed in it, so that you don't notice a friend / partner speak to you? Or started reading a novel and before you know it you have lost contact with time - time has flown by in what felt like a short space of time? How about when you've been driving a familiar route and suddenly you arrive at your destination but you don't really remember parts of the journey? These are all examples of naturally occurring trans states or hypnosis, but in the example of driving a car you would immediately switch into a conscious state and avoid danger if a car pulled out in front of you!

To de-mystify it, hypnobirthing is a simple antenatal preparation for birth that involves:

- self-hypnosis;
- easy to learn techniques to work with your breath;
- guided relaxations;
- an understanding about the power of the mind-body connection;
- developing an understanding about the powerful effect of language on the mind and body during labour;
- positive affirmations;
- understanding the power of hormones released during natural labour and the birth environment during labour;
- informed decision making and an understanding of your options and choices during labour and birth;
- learning how to release fears;
- learning about how the body works during labour and birth and what factors can help or hinders this process (some of these factors we have already covered in previous chapters).

So, hypnobirthing is a complete antenatal education and preparation in and of itself, combined with some very practical elements. It might be useful to think of it as a mindset-reset or overhaul.

An essential part of a hypnobirthing course (and any good antenatal course or preparation for birth book) is the process where you learn practical skills to use to enable you to remain calm and relaxed during your labour and birth, combined with knowledge and informed decision to enable your birth to be a positive experience.

Women who practice hypnobirthing frequently report that they are able to relax and enjoy their pregnancy more and feel more positive preparing for labour and birth. They enjoy listening to the guided relaxations, fall asleep listening to the MP3s and learn to trust their bodies. Women already know how to give birth, but sadly, it is common that faith and trust in the process has been lost along the way. Hypnobirthing gives women and their birth partners a set of tools and techniques that can help them to use their already present, natural birthing instincts.

The specific practice of breathing techniques and changed mindset can often result in a more comfortable birthing experience, with couples reporting that they felt more calm and in control, however their birth unfolds. Hypnobirthing has become very popular, with many women using the techniques and some Midwives and Maternity Units offering classes.

Hypnobirthing is not necessarily about removing pain, but rather, it is about reframing it and understanding how your body is working to birth your baby. The breathing and mindset practices help to allow you to let go, give yourself over to your body rather than fighting against or resisting the contractions, which reduces or eliminates fear and panic, with all the problems that they bring.

Whilst some women report that they only experienced tightenings or pressure during their labour, other women report that they did feel some pain, but did not feel out of control or frightened by it, understanding what its purpose of each contraction was and relaxing as much as possible with each surge, maintaining their focus so that it would not spiral out of control.

If you decide to undertake a hypnobirthing course, it is best to start earlier in the pregnancy rather than later, with most couples starting between 20-30 weeks of pregnancy. This is to enable lots of repetition in order to embrace a different mindset around birth. However if you come to hypnobirthing later than 30 weeks, it is important not to be put off – you will just need to commit yourself and intensify your practice, rather than building it up slowly.

Advantages of hypnobirthing

Hypnobirthing techniques help a woman to relax, which in turn:

- Means that she is going to be breathing deeply and calmly, which increases oxygen to herself and her baby.
- Means she will be activating the parasympathetic response of 'calm and connection' ensuring the uterus, placenta and baby will have a good blood supply.
- Surges or contractions are likely to be more efficient.
- The 'fight or flight' mechanism is not stimulated.
- Endorphin production, the body's natural and super powerful painkiller, is enhanced.
- Women and partners feel involved and empowered.
- Birth partners are very much involved and have an important role.
- It is common that no medication is needed.
- Women are informed and understand how their body works in labour.
- Women report feeling calm and in control, whatever turn their birth takes.
- There are no harmful side effects to the mother or baby – in fact babies benefit from the increased oxygen from the calm, regular, deep breathing.
- Practising hypnobirthing during pregnancy will often mean that the woman is able to feel more positive approaching the labour and birth. She will have a tool kit to enable her to deal with challenges or 'wobbly' moments, which means that she is able to enjoy her pregnancy without unnecessary fears hanging over her.

Potential disadvantages of hypnobirthing:

- Consistent time and effort is required in order to get the full benefits of hypnobirthing – but this is often described as relaxing, enjoyable and positive, so is this really a disadvantage?
- Doing a hypnobirthing course costs money, but many women successfully can practice hypnobirthing by reading books and listening to the relaxation MP3s.
- You may not have a practitioner in your area – but a Skype class may be an option.
- Sometimes women feel it didn't work for them, or that it only helped them for part of their labour and feel disappointed about this.

What is hypnosis?

Many people think hypnosis is a mysterious thing that someone does to them. They may picture a person lying on a couch, with the hypnotherapist beside them working their magic while the patient is passive. In actual fact, all hypnosis is self-hypnosis, and no one can make you do anything you do not want to do in hypnosis.

"There are a number of definitions of hypnosis. It a natural, though altered, state of mind. We all enter some form of hypnosis several times a day, like when we are driving and pass a turn-off because our mind is wandering. We can also go into the state of hypnosis when engrossed in a film or TV show. Additionally, everyone goes through natural, altered states before falling asleep, and while awakening. Therefore, most people can enter hypnotic relaxation easily, provided they want to, and provided they feel comfortable doing so." (Hunter, R 2015)

The mind is incredibly complex, but try thinking of it as existing in two parts: the conscious and subconscious mind. The conscious mind regulates decision-making, processing of information, perception through the five senses, critical thinking, analytical thinking, spacial awareness, judgements, awareness of self and awareness of time. The subconscious mind regulates memory, imagination, dreaming and instinct, and it relays information back to the conscious.

What happens during hypnosis is that when a person enters hypnosis they become relaxed and the critical part of the brain, which allows us all to distinguish between what is real and what is imaginary, moves out of the way temporarily and allows the conscious mind to become open to positive ideas and suggestions. This allows the subconscious mind, which does not distinguish between what is real and what is imaginary to become open to all sorts of positive realities, such as 'you are a non-smoker', or *'you are prepared and ready to relax into a wonderful birth experience'*.

Roughly speaking, when a person becomes relaxed in hypnosis, the critical part of the brain, which allows you to tell the difference between what is real and what is imaginary, moves out of the way and allows the conscious mind to quieten. This allows the subconscious mind (which doesn't distinguish between what is real or unreal) to be able to accept all sorts of positive realities, such as 'you are a non-smoker', or 'you are no longer afraid of spiders' or *'you are prepared and ready to relax into a wonderful birth experience'*.

A person must be willing and interested, as only they can allow themselves to lie down, begin deep breathing, to relax and listen to the guided relaxations. No one can make them use their imagination to visualise certain events.

It is good that hypnosis is voluntary, which means that you are always completely in control of yourself, but it does also mean a person needs to genuinely be interested in giving hypnobirthing a go and making a commitment to using the power of the mind. Hypnobirthing would be useless if you had no interest or belief in it.

Some people say, after they have used self-hypnosis or visited a hypnotherapist, 'It can't have worked as I was aware of what was going on around me the whole time, I heard the phone ring and people talking outside'. However, self-hypnosis simply means having quiet, undisturbed time, focussing inwardly, or on a particular subject, and allowing yourself to drift into a deeply relaxed state of mind, possibly hearing your partner read out one of the scripts in this book, or listening to the MP3s in a positive and repetitive way. In hypnosis you are still aware of what is going on around you, but open to positive suggestions and less focussed on your immediate surroundings.

To use hypnobirthing requires you to practice the techniques. Most of us have grown up thinking of labour and birth as something that we have to 'get through', and that it will be incredibly painful and frightening. We've heard our auntie's, our mother's and our friends' birth stories, not to mention how birth is portrayed in the media and on TV shows, and so unless you're very fortunate, it's usually pretty negative stories.

Parents often report they enjoy a little time out a few times a week to focus on the pregnancy, baby and each other. A woman can also practice alone and falling asleep to the MP3s is fine.

To unlearn these unhelpful programmes, stories and beliefs we have about birth takes time and repetition and setting aside a little time in your week to focus on this. When actions and ideas are repeated over and over they become habits and beliefs which can be very powerful.

In a previous chapter we talked about the subconscious as a 'library', perhaps with a negative birth section. Self-hypnosis is one way to clear that out and fill that section with positivity instead. Then, when you go into labour, your mind will access the positive birth information you've shelved in your subconscious. Your brain will believe that 'birth is OK and safe', which can prevent the fear-pain-cycle and raised adrenalin levels negatively affecting your natural release of helpful birth hormones.

When a labouring woman is relaxed, her surges or contractions can do the job they are meant to do. This means that her uterine muscles work together as nature intended – the upper segment of the uterus contracts strongly and with each successive contraction the muscle fibres of the upper segment become shorter and thicker (retraction) which in turn draws the weaker, thinner part of the lower uterus up and in doing so this dilates the cervix, gradually moving the baby downwards. With each contraction the upper part of the uterus becomes thicker and thicker. Tension in the mind and body causes the cervix to remain taut and closed, meaning that the two sets of muscles work against each other, which may result in an increased experience of pain and a slower labour.

Releasing Fear

Being able to release fears is a big part of hypnobirthing which has been covered in a previous chapter. When you listen to a negative birth story you add to or top up your birth 'birth mind library' with yet more negative stories. It may not seem like much at the time, but you can't unhear things that are said and your subconscious mind remembers it all. Now is the time to be solely focusing on preparing for a positive birth. Rather than watching the news last thing at night, which is usually a less than relaxing experience, you could instead choose to listen to your hypnobirthing MP3 (all the scripts later in this chapter are available to you as MP3s). You could watch a positive birth video (you'll find carefully selected ones at www.baby-bumps.net), read some positive birth stories (there are some at the end of this chapter) or join a hypnobirthing Facebook page such as *Baby Bumps – Hypnobirthing South London* to have your news feed full of positive, supportive birth stories and information.

Rather than watching the news last thing at night, which is usually a less than relaxing experience, instead listen to your hypnobirthing MP3 (all the scripts later in this chapter are available to you as MP3s).

Watch a positive birth video (you'll find carefully selected ones at www.baby-bumps.net), read some positive birth stories (there are some at the end of this chapter) or join a hypnobirthing Facebook page such as *Baby Bumps – Hypnobirthing South London* to have your news feed full of supportive, positive birth stories and information.

Think about where your fears come from – are they actually your fears or just things that you have heard along the way? Birth is very safe for most women, but we tend to only remember the negative things we hear.

Write your concerns down, whether they are about birth or anything else that you want to release. Ask yourself "how likely is this to happen?", "is this my truth, or is it someone else's story?" If 'XYZ' is truly is on the cards for you, ask yourself "who can I talk to in order to gain some perspective on it all?" Sometimes the action of simply writing your fears down and/or talking it through with someone you trust, is enough to get it out of your head and make it feel a little less overwhelming.

If you still feel after honestly thinking about your fears, that they are very real for you, focus a lot of time on listening to the fear release script/MP3 in this chapter and listen to this above the others until you start to feel a shift or change. You can also read other hypnobirthing books and saturate your brain with as many different sources of positive birth stories as is possible! If at all possible, attend a hypnobirthing course.

Consider seeing an experienced hypnotherapist if you feel that none of the above is helping you or you still feel stuck in fear.

Breathing

It may sound obvious, and we've talked about this a lot already, but using specific breathing techniques during labour & birth is *the* most important tool. If you were to get one thing 'down pat' for the day, working effectively with your breath is that one thing. It's literally foundational for a calm and as-relaxed-as-is-possible birth and it is pretty much impossible to panic when you are breathing slowly and rhythmically.

Not only that, it's a great life skill to be able to go within yourself and calm yourself quickly using just your breath. I still use my breathing techniques to this day, almost 10 years on from when I did my hypnobirthing course when expecting my second child.

There are many different types of breathing techniques out there to learn, but you only need to keep it simple – a long, slow breath in through your nose, gently released out through a relaxed mouth & jaw - think of it as 'baby breathing' – you are breathing in very deeply & slowly so that your oxygen fuelled breath isn't just filling your lungs but you are breathing into your belly and down to your baby too, giving them space and oxygen and then releasing the breath out alongside with any stress and tension you feel. You can, if you want to, couple your breathing with visualisations which we will cover later in this chapter and some of which have already been mentioned.

Pre surge body scan:

Try to relax as soon as you feel the next surge starting to build. Greet it with a slow out breath or sigh and do a mental scan of your body from top to toe. Is your brow furrowed? Soften it. Are your eyes scrunched up, relax them. Is your jaw clenched? Gently open it and relax it. Are your shoulders scrunched up around your ears? Drop them down. Open and relax your palms.

This literally only takes a moment to do and releasing all tension as you feel the surge building allows your mind and body to be ready to take it on! You might like to imagine a wave or waterfall of relaxation starting at the top of your head and going all the way down to your toes, removing any tension as it passes through you, out and down into the ground. Remember, the surge will only last for around a minute.

If whilst being aware of the power of the contraction, you are able to relax your jaw and make your whole body relaxed and limp, breathing deeply and gently, fear will not arise. Talk to your birth partner about where you usually hold tension in your body and ask them to remind you to relax those areas. For example, if the shoulders are your natural area of tension as your surge begins, your birth partner can keep an eye out for this. They can then remind you to release and drop them down, perhaps gently pressing down on them or stroking, and using a key word you've agreed (see the 'Top to Toe' relaxation) such as 'relax', 'release', 'soften' or 'let go'. Practicing this in advance will give it more meaning on the day and will help your partner to know what to look out for and what words may help you to release tension.

Remember, all that you need to do is to handle one surge or contraction at a time.

Using visualisations when breathing

Some women may find it helpful to visualise what the body is doing when breathing calmly during labour. During the first stage the cervix is softening and opening, moving the baby down. As you breathe during the first stage of labour, you could think of visualisations such as standing in a beautiful open meadow feeling the soft grass on your feet. Or picturing a flower's petals slowly opening and blooming. If you prefer, you can visualise your cervix softening, shortening and opening easily to let your baby begin his journey out.

The second stage of labour is all about your baby's passage into the world as he or she moves downwards with each surge. For the second stage you might imagine your baby being nudged downwards by your powerful out breath. It can help to focus the out breath down the back of your throat (in a similar way to the Ujjayi breath for anyone who does yoga) and see your baby in your mind's eye moving peacefully down with each out breath. You may like to imagine your out breath pushing downwards like a coffee plunger, encouraging your baby to do the same.

Below are some of the advantages to learning breathing techniques for labour & birth:

- Increased oxygen levels for you and your baby
- Helps keeps you calm and clear headed no matter what
- Gives you something to focus on *right now*
- Lowers your heart rate
- Stabilises blood pressure
- Conserves your energy during labour
- Relieves stress
- Stops panic breathing and breath holding, which make you feel light headed and out of control
- Can be coupled with counting, affirmations and visualisations to make it even more powerful and effective

As mentioned in the chapter on breathing, it may be helpful to count how many slow, relaxed breaths you normally take during a minute. As you know, a surge or contraction, lasts around one minute, which is normally around 10 – 14 long, slow, relaxed breaths; at its peak, when the surge is at its strongest, this is around 4 – 5 lovely breaths (around 45 seconds). You can do anything for 45 seconds!

It's important to realise that learning breathing techniques is not only for the labouring woman, but also the birth partner can benefit from using them to keep them relaxed and calm on the day. Encourage your birth partner to practice as well.

- Increases oxygen to you and your baby
- Keeps you calm and clear headed no matter what
- Gives you something to focus on *right now*
- Lowers your heart rate
- Stabilises blood pressure
- Conserves energy

- Improves circulation
- Relieves stress and adrenalin
- Relaxation techniques such as breathing are linked to a reduced chance of having an assisted birth (forceps or ventouse)
- Stops panic breathing and breath holding, which make you feel light headed and out of control
- Can be coupled with counting, affirmations and visualisations to make it even more powerful and useful

You might like to go back and re-read the chapter about breathing techniques and try out some of the ideas discussed there. Use the breathing and positive affirmations and other MP3s plus the scripts included with this book to get your practice in! It's important to remember not to be disheartened if you find that you're not able to get the out breath very long when you start practicing – this will improve with practice and repetition.

Like all the techniques, this isn't something you'd do a few times and expect it to work on the day. It's a skill that you are learning in order to be able to relax despite feeling the intensity of the surges, and like most skills, it takes practice and repetition before it feels second nature.

Informed Decision Making

Labour and birth don't always go as expected and it's useful to keep a flexible outlook on it. Having said that, writing a birth preferences/birth plan is very important as it enables you to start thinking about your wishes for your birth and what you might want in other situations should your birth take a different turn. There is an example of a birth plan in this book.

Sometimes, during the course of a labour an unexpected complication may arise and your Midwife may suggest a way to proceed. Your midwife may ask how you feel about 'X, Y or Z' and it can be hard to know how best to go forward. It is, absolutely fine to let the Midwife know what your birth preferences are, and providing it is not an emergency situation (and it will be obvious if it is), you can ask as many questions as you want to. Asking questions can help you to gather information, feel involved and make informed decisions, rather than making decisions based around fear and the unknown, or feeling pushed into a decision without fully understanding it.

Different Midwives have different approaches and, as wonderful as Midwives are, they are only human and, like the rest of us, possibly have a preferred way of doing something – but there may be another way of achieving the same result, whatever it may be. It is always worthwhile asking questions. Below are some suggestions:

"What alternative is there to 'X' – are there any other options we could consider?"

"How might what you're suggesting affect me/my partner and our baby?"

"Would you please explain that a bit more as I don't understand fully?"

"Is my partner/baby OK?"

- and remember to use the BRAIN decision making tool.

Informed decision making makes for a positive birth! A woman and her partner who felt that they were able to ask relevant questions, get information and understand fully before agreeing to something will more likely feel empowered. This is such an important issue – it can potentially change the course of your experience during labour and birth, by how listened to and respected you feel during your birth, just by being fully involved and asking a few simple questions. During labour, you can ask for 5 minutes alone to think through what is being suggested, without someone hovering over you waiting for an immediate answer.

Tips on including your hypnobirthing practice in your everyday life:

Schedule it in. Literally set aside time. For example; on a Tuesday, Thursday & Sunday for 20 minutes you do one of the couple's relaxations/scripts or some massage practice whilst dinner is cooking. If you tag it onto the end of the day chances are you'll be too tired & sleepy after dinner to do it or say 'we'll do it tomorrow instead'. And tomorrow will come… and go… with nothing achieved, again. So deliberately set time aside.

Build it up slowly, then increase it as you get closer to your due date. If you have plenty of time then doing some practice three times a week is great. If you are short of time or the due date is looming, then increase the practice more. You'll never look back & say 'we did way too much practice, we were far too prepared!'

Play your positive affirmations MP3 while you're getting ready for work, in the bath, preparing dinner, pottering about, and so on. Actively listen to it and also tune out too. It is all going in and doing a whole lot of good.

Fall asleep to the guided relaxations. Whilst the Fear-Release MP3 is best listened to actively (though don't worry if you fall asleep – enjoy the rest as you must have needed it!) as it gives you the opportunity to blast away your concerns, the other MP3s can be listened to in bed and it is more than OK if you fall asleep. It is all going into your subconscious mind, helping to turn any unhelpful negative programming on its head. When you are on maternity leave, listening to the MP3s is a great way to take a day time nap too – to be able to fall asleep, feeling confident and ready for your labour and birth is great.

Read some or all of this book & others together as a couple. One couple on a course I facilitated told me they would read a chapter of the book each in bed, out loud to one another, which I thought was a lovely way to read the book and both share the information.

Watch a birth video once a week – Watching a positive birth video can be a powerful antidote to all the negative, dramatic rubbish we see on TV about birth.

Daily breathing and visualisation practice. It may be easy to breathe deeply and calmly now, but when in you are in advanced labour, if you have not done any breathing practice, it is harder to relax on command. Slow, rhythmic breathing is the basic foundation to a calm birth and will keep you clear headed and feeling in control. It's also super useful postnatally. It really is a fantastic life skill to calm yourself down by using just a few breaths!

We have already talked about visualisation, but as a reminder, spend time visualising your birth – see yourself arriving at your place of birth (or see the home birth midwife arriving at your home). Add in lots of detail. Visualise the end of your labour when you are holding your baby, feeling amazing and proud! This is a lovely thing to do before you fall asleep at night or when sat waiting for something like in a traffic jam or when waiting for the train to work.

Create a birth board with wedding photos/couple's photos, scan photos, holiday photos, affirmations & positive birth quotes (all written in the present tense). If a birth board isn't your thing, then simply stick your positive affirmations and

...ll over your home on post it notes. It might not sound like much, but noticing them, reading them and repeating them will make a difference. It's all about the repetition.

Schedule it in! Seriously, you will not regret having put the effort in. It really makes all the difference when a couple/woman has done regular practice. You won't get a second chance to birth your baby so give it all you've got!

Suggestions on how to use your hypnobirthing when in labour:

You've read this book, maybe you also completed a hypnobirthing course and focused on the all important practice. Your baby is on his way now, so how should you use your hypnobirthing techniques? What do you do when?

The good thing about hypnobirthing is that there are no rules. You have learned a toolbox of techniques to pick and choose from. Some you will likely prefer to others and find them more relaxing and beneficial.

Below are some suggestions for each stage of labour.

Early Labour:

You may wake in the night feeling your contractions start. Many midwives say 'don't wake your partner, let them rest' – I'm not sure any woman has ever actually done this!

If you can, go back to sleep. Exciting as it is, labour is usually quite a slow, long process. If you cannot sleep perhaps have something to eat, a bath then curl up in bed, warm and dark (use an eye mask if needed) and have your partner read out one of the scripts. If you're lucky you could fall asleep, if not, you will feel grounded and calm and you can just rest.

Once awake, or if you're unable to fall asleep, try to carry on business as usual for as long as possible. So if it's the middle of the night put on one of your MP3s and rest with your eyes shut and your phone on aeroplane mode or on silent at least.

If it's daytime and surges/contractions are still mild and infrequent, go out for a walk or for something to eat. Put on a box set, something that will make you laugh. Eat, drink, bounce on your birth ball.

Go for a walk but also rest so you don't tire yourself out. Consider making a meal for your return. Tidy up so you return to a clear house. You may think these suggestions sound crazy, but for many women surges are very mild in early labour and you'd be far better off distracting yourself and ignoring them for as long as is possible.

Don't worry about timing the surges until they are requiring all of your focus and attention and you don't want to talk through them. Have your positive affirmations MP3 or one of the other MP3s playing in the background or on headphones. Their familiarity will be comforting to you.

Gentle stroking or massage may be good now. You might like your partner to read you a script. And you enjoy baths, snacks or sips of water.

Active Labour:

Once things are in full flow you will find it useful to start focusing on your breathing. Massage may or may not be of interest. Your partner can now start to time your surges – there are many apps out there to help with this if that's easier.

Words of encouragement from your partner for in between surges.

Time to go in:

Earphones at the ready and MP3 on in the car/taxi if you want to really stay in the zone. If your partner can sit with you in the back all the better. Perhaps they could read one of the scripts out to you. If it's bright outside you could put on some sunglasses and if you don't want to listen to a MP3 you can listen to music as a distraction, or use ear plugs if you want to shut out the world completely.

Arrive in hospital & meet your midwife. Partners will ensure your birth plan gets read.

Get all the lights down, listen to a whole script from your partner or put your MP3 on. All of these things will ground you as you've listened and practiced with them for so long during your pregnancy. Just hearing your partner with their familiar voice saying words you know so well will help to relax & calm you.

Lower the bed and use it as a prop to lean on whilst sitting on a birth ball. Your breathing will be of great use now.

Transition:

This part of labour can feel intense for many women and it's very common to have feelings of self doubt now. Remember it's the shortest part though and the co-breathing will be useful if you feel like you're feeling tense, holding your breath or are aware of feeling panicky.

Time to meet your baby:

Once you are ready to breathe/push your baby out, keep those lovely oxygen fuelled breaths coming, sending your breath downwards to nudge your baby out. Consider your position and remember how the pelvis looked when a woman was flat on her back, how it leads to a restriction in space and how helpful gravity is.

Now that your baby has finally arrived, darkness, skin to skin, keeping warm, emptying your bladder and being upright will help the placenta to come out easily.

Postnatally you can continue to use your breathing techniques as being able to relax at will is a fabulous tool to have learned!

Hypnobirthing Scripts:

All of the scripts and affirmations are available as MP3 downloads, included in the purchase of this book so you can listen to them alone, if you wake up in the night and are struggling to get back to sleep, on maternity leave, to have on in the background and during labour. There is one for birth partners too. To access all MP3s visit this link: **www.baby-bumps.net/bookmp3s**. All scripts have been checked by a qualified clinical hypnotherapist for accuracy, safety and quality.

As it can be lovely to have your partner read them to you too, the wording on each MP3 is below. If you like, your partner can include an arm stroke, hand hold/stroke or neck/shoulder stroke in with the script reading. If you do this stroking each time he or she reads you a script or you listen to a MP3 together this form of touch will act as a trigger to remind you of feeling confidence and trust around birth. You can then use this on the day at any point in your labour either on its own or combined with words.

: feels a bit strange at first reading these scripts
ely be some laughter initially! Eventually
past this and find yourself looking forward to

Birth partners – when you read out a relaxation script, try and
keep your voice soft and slow, with plenty of well placed
pauses.

Breathing practice & positive affirmations MP3:

Breathing during your labour and birth:

*Remember not to be disheartened if you're unable to get very deep,
long breaths at first. The more you practice this the easier it will get.
Just follow your own, comfortable pattern of breathing.*

By the time you are ready to give birth, your uterus will be the
biggest, strongest muscle in your entire body. For it to work well
and with ease, it needs a good oxygen supply and good blood
supply.

During your labour you can help your uterus do its amazing job
well with slow, rhythmic breathing. Not only will this keep you
feeling super calm and in control, it will also provide your uterus
with all it needs to make each surge powerful and efficient.

It's all about the rhythm. Rhythmic breathing, rhythmic words,
rhythmic movement.

Let's try a few breathing techniques out now.

Before we start, take a moment to breathe in and sigh any tension
out and make your whole body floppy and relaxed. This can also
be helpful to do when you are in labour, as you feel your next
surge building.

So go ahead, a deep breath in.... and sigh out softly, releasing all stress and tension easily.

Breathing technique 1.

Counted breathing.

In a moment, take a big breath in through your nose and softly sigh the breath out, trying to make the out breath a little longer than the in breath. Keep your shoulders relaxed and your jaw soft.

Ready? OK. Breathing in, 2, 3, 4 and out 2....3....4....5.....6
Let's try another one – Breathing in, 2, 3, 4 and out
2....3....4....5.....6

And do the last two in your own time now, following your own comfortable pattern of breathing. (pause to allow)

Breathing technique 2:

Visualisation.

Close your eyes and think of a colour that makes you feel calm and confident. Just pick the first colour that comes into your mind.

Now you have that colour in your mind, keep your eyes closed and see that colour in front of you in all its vibrancy and beauty.

In a moment try taking a deep breath in and inhale this strong, calm colour in through your nose, fill your lungs with this colour and finally feel it swirl around your baby, calming your baby as it does.

Now sigh out the colour, with a soft relaxed jaw, and see it spreading far out in front of you, perhaps like when you're able to see your breath on a very cold day. See the colour slowly drift away, taking any tension along with it.

So you're going to breath in the colour, a long, slow, deep breath then sigh it out softly – seeing it drift away, taking all tension with it.

Now in your own time, try this visualisation breath three times.

(Pause long enough plus a bit more, for 3 more long deep breaths.)

Breathing technique 3.

Mantras.

Mantras are simply positive sayings. Repeating words in your head or softly out loud will give you focus and add to the rhythm in your body and mind.

You can of course make your own up but if you don't have one in mind, in a moment, try one of these whilst you practise 3 more slow, deep, calming breaths:

I breathe in relaxation..... I sigh out softness
I breathe in calm.... I release tension
In strength... out love ...

So go ahead, try out 3 more breaths with the mantra or mantras of your choice. (pause to allow her to do this)

And finally, take another deep breath in and on the soft sighing-out breath try slowly and calmly saying relax, relax, relax

Each day at the start and end of the day spend a few moments practising these breathing techniques. Try with your eyes closed, bringing your focus inwards, and with your eyes open.

Positive affirmations for labour and birth:

I give birth easily and calmly.

My birth is smooth and comfortable.

I believe I can and so I will.

Each breath and surge brings my baby closer to me.

Women all over the world are giving birth with me.

Breathing deeply and slowly relaxes my muscles, making my labour comfortable.

My body knows how to birth my baby, just as it knew how to grow my baby.

I am strong and I trust my body knows what to do.

I relax into each surge, maximising oxygen to me and my baby.

I keep gently active, I create space for my baby to be born swiftly and easily.

*Surges are powerful and strong, but they are not stronger then me because they **are** me.*

I am using my surges to birth my baby.

I relax and let my body take over to birth my baby.

I breathe in relaxation, I breathe out softness.

As labour progresses my relaxation deepens and my body softens and opens easily.

Whatever turn my birth takes, I remain calm and in control.

I am able to make decisions about my birth clearly and calmly.

I am ready and looking forward to the birth of my baby.

All is well.

Fear-Release script:

I'd like you to get comfortable and close your eyes and allow your breathing to slow down and become relaxed and smooth. As you breathe, in... and out... you start to feel your body relax and sink comfortably down. It feels lovely to give yourself a little time out to relax like this.

And now, in your own time, take three deep, slow breaths in... and out.... and with each out breath you start to feel any tension drop away and flow easily out of you. **(pause to observe your partner doing 2-3 slow breaths)**

Now you're starting to feel so relaxed we can focus on deepening this further through your entire body, from tip to toe. Starting at the top, you relax and soften your forehead..... relax your eyes, feeling any tension in and around your eyes being washed away.... feel your jaw and tongue relax.... With your face now relaxed and free of all tension.

Let the muscles in your neck relax. Allow your shoulders to sink down a bit more with each out breath. Feel this lovely calmness spread down through your chest and down into your arms. Your hands and even your fingertips are now relaxed and loose.

Feel your stomach relax.... your pelvis....A heavy, soft feeling of wonderful relaxation now travels down the tops of your legs, through your knees, down to your lower legs and now reaches your feet and toes.

Pause for a moment now and if you note any areas of tension that may have crept back in, release it all gently now. Every last bit of tension is now draining out of your body and mind so you can enjoy this restful feeling.

Now I'd like you to picture something like a volume dial or dimmer switch with 3 notches on it, from 3 to zero. In a moment we're going to enjoy 3 slow, calming breaths and as you release tension on the out breath you see the switch or the dial turn down a notch, helping you to sink down further into relaxation. So go ahead and take 3 breaths in and out, allowing your relaxation to easily deepen with each out breath and with each dial down. **(pause to allow 3 breaths)** Now you are on zero and are very relaxed indeed.

Your entire body feels heavy, warm, soft and completely free of tension. Just enjoy this feeling for a moment or two. **(pause)**

Now that you are feeling calm and at ease, I am going to talk you through a gentle, guided relaxation. If you need to cough or move or stretch just go ahead. If you notice your mind wandering during the relaxation just gently guide it back to my voice.

Any sounds that break in such as voices outside or a phone ringing or cars passing by will just send you into a deeper relaxation, so just let these sounds drift on through you.

OK so I want you to use your imagination and see yourself walking towards a beautiful beach, it can be a beach you know, or it can be an imagined beach, in your mind.

It's a lovely day and the temperature is just right. Feel the warm breeze gently blowing across your face and skin. Take a deep breath in and smell the fresh sea air. You feel so happy to be here at this peaceful and special place.

This area is completely safe, and apart from a few people far away in the distance it's just you here.

You walk down a pathway leading to the soft sandy beach. You are enjoying the quietness of the beach. You can hear the gentle, rhythmic sound of the sea rolling in.... and out.... Such a calm and lovely place to be.

You arrive at some steps leading down to the beach. You take your shoes off and feel the warm, sandy steps beneath your bare feet. There are 10 steps down, and as I count you down, with each step you feel more and more relaxed

, with every step you take.

10... 9.... – pausing for a moment, breathing deeply, smelling the sea air, feeling relaxed.... 8... 7... you feel your feet on the warm steps... . notice how relaxed you now feel. 6... 5..., each step down brings with it more relaxation.... 4.... 3.... your relaxation is becoming deeper and deeper. 2... you feel so relaxed, comfortable and at peace. And 1, you are now on the beach, feet sinking into the warm sand, feeling so calm.

You decide to walk down to the water's edge. You watch the soft waves rolling into the shore. The air smells wonderfully fresh. You look out over the water, far into the horizon. The clear blue sky looks beautiful against the green-blue sea. This beautiful place always makes you feel totally relaxed and at ease.

Now imagine yourself walking a short way away from the shore onto the warm sandy beach where you lay out your towel and drop your shoes onto the sand and sit down.

Next to you is a small wooden boat with a rope attached to the front. This is a special boat which has the capacity to take away all worries and concerns.

Pause for a moment now, and consider any concerns you have, these could be about labour, birth or anything at all that is worrying you. **(pause to allow images to come up)**

And now taking your time, see yourself either mentally or physically putting each and every one of these worries or concerns into the little wooden boat. Whatever you think each worry looks like I want you to see yourself putting it inside the boat. It could be words, images or just mentally imagining it... Take a few moments now and pile all of the worries into the boat feeling lighter as each worry leaves your body and mind. **(pause to allow this to take place)**

Now that all of your worries are piled in the small wooden boat, you stand up, pick up the rope and pull the small boat the few steps towards the shore.

Now you're at the edge of the shore, you give the boat a firm push into the sea. The current takes the boat out into the sea. You watch the boat drift further and further away. The boat with all your worries inside it becomes smaller and smaller and smaller, until it is a tiny dot in the distance.... and then it completely disappears from your sight, taking all your concerns with it, each and every worry gone forever.

Standing at the shore, you take a deep breath in, and out.... and you feel so light and free, happy and relaxed.

Enjoying your new worry-free self you walk back to your towel, lie down and feel the warm rays of the glorious sunshine on your skin.

The warm sunshine and the rhythmic sound of the waves makes you feel even more drowsy and relaxed – in fact you are feeling more relaxed and peaceful than you have for a very long time.

You take a moment to imagine and visualise how calm and relaxed your baby's birth will be, who will be there supporting you, where you will be, and how confident and at ease you will feel. **PAUSE.**

Now focus on your baby's arrival and see you both together, everything went as you hoped for. The atmosphere is calm and your baby is in your arms, sleeping peacefully. Feel your baby's heavy, warm weight in your arms. You are both so happy and content that everything went just as you visualised it. **Pause**

So it's now time to leave the beach, feeling assured, light and free of worry. You know this confidence and relaxation that you have created is here to stay throughout your pregnancy, your baby's birth and beyond.

You love how confident you feel. So calm, so rested, so energised. You feel strong and in control. You know all is well.

If you have fallen asleep and have no need to wake up, just continue your restful sleep. Should you need to get up and continue with your day you can now start walking back towards the steps.

I will now count your steps back up. On the tenth step you will come back to the present feeling excited, confident and so ready for your baby's birth.

One, two three, feeling the energy in your arms and legs. Four, five, six, you gently stretch, feeling revitalised. 7 and 8, you take a deep breath in and feel yourself becoming more alert. 9 you are now coming back to present time feeling happy and knowing all is well. And 10, open your eyes feeling alert, calm and in control.

Top to Toe Tension Release

Practising this longer tension release now will help you be able to do a quicker, more efficient pre-surge body scan. Let your partner know which word you chose at the end of the relaxation so they know what it is and you can let them know when it might help them to say it to you – perhaps at the beginning or end of a surge.

Sit comfortably or lay down. Bring your attention to your breathing, don't try to alter it, just pay attention to it for a moment.

Now focus on your physical body – where are you feeling tension or tightness? Just notice where it is held in your body for now.

OK now let's start to release all tension from your body, tip to toe, using your breath. Bringing soothing relaxation to you on the inhalation and releasing any tension on the out breath.

If your mind wanders throughout this relaxation just bring it back to your breath and the body part you want to focus on. During the relaxation simply follow your own comfortable breathing pattern so nothing feels forced. I will leave a pause long enough for you to do each breath twice, if you want to.

Gently close your eyes and focus on the top of your head for a moment. Take a slow easy breath in and on the out breath, release any tension here, feeling this whole area relax. (pause)

Now move down to your forehead. Breathe in... and when you breath out imagine your brow softly smoothing out. Starting to relax now. (pause)

160

Bring your attention to your eyes. Focus on all the tiny muscles in and around your eyes. Breathe in and on the out breath feel your eyes relax, relax, relax. (pause)

Focus on the lower part of your face – your cheeks, lips and jaw. Breathing in, and on the out breath let your cheeks relax and your jaw and lips soften. You may find your mouth slightly opens as you relax. Feel any tension drifting away. (pause)

Good.

Now move on down to the back of your neck. Breathe in and let the out breath carry away any stress and tightness you have in this area. (pause)

Focus on your shoulders and the top of your back. On the in breath gently raise your shoulders up and release them down on the out breath – all tension releasing as they heavily and naturally sink down. (pause)

Notice how calm you feel and how your breathing has slowed.

Feeling super relaxed and peaceful.

Bring your attention to your arms and hands now. Breathe in and on the out breath feel your arms becoming heavy and limp - all tension releasing out released through your fingertips. (pause)

Focus on your stomach and mid-lower back. Tune into your baby – whether they are active or sleeping, he or she is enjoying this wonderful calmness you're giving them. Spend a few breaths now relaxing this area, sending love to your baby and feel yourself drifting into a deep relaxation with every out breath. (longer pause to allow for several breaths).

And now your bottom, pelvis and hips. Let go of tightness and tension held here with your out breath, sigh it all out. (pause)

Good.

Finally your legs to the way to the tips of your toes. Breathe in, and on the out breath feel every last bit of stress releasing all the way down your legs, down through your knees, to your ankles and out through your toes.

Your body is now relaxed from head to toe.

Think of a word which represents this relaxation that you have just created. It could be 'calm', 'relax', 'peace', 'safe' 'serenity' 'release' or something else — whatever word you decide on just repeat it to yourself in your head or out loud for a few moments. (Pause to allow for this). That's great.

You know how strong you are, your body and mind work together to safely, easily and comfortably bring your baby to you at the perfect time for you both. And each time you say your chosen word out loud or to yourself you will bring to you all this effortless relaxation which you have created. All you need to do is breathe in and on the out breath say your word and all tension will swiftly release from the top of your head all the way down to your toes to be taken away and replaced with calm.

And now it's time to come back to the present.... If you've fallen asleep and have no need to rise, enjoy a deep, restful sleep. Otherwise, slowly become aware of your fingers and toes... your eyelids starting to feel lighter... Feeling the weight of your body fully now... and when you're ready, open your eyes and continue with your day feeling calm, confident and prepared for your baby's birth.

Garden Relaxation - Mother

This relaxation was written for the mother, with the birth partner's version to follow.

*The fourth paragraph below, in italics: when your partner reads this out to you if you wish to you can personalise this and change the garden scene to a favourite holiday beach walk, or a familiar woodland walk you like to do, etc.

Just settle yourself into the most comfortable position and allow your eyes to gently close now......you don't have to stay absolutely still, but it may be that that's all you actually want to do......just to allow yourself to settle more and more deeply into the chair or on the bed....

Now take a deep breath in..... and let it out slowly......and allow yourself to become more relaxed as you do so......as though you are breathing away all tensions from your mind and body......

Now bring your attention to your breathing and allow your breathing to slow down and deepen...... as you breathe in, imagine calmness and relaxation going in....and as you breathe out each time, imagine tension drifting away from you.....

*For a moment or two I wonder if you can imagine yourself walking in the most beautiful, peaceful garden.....a place where you feel completely comfortable, relaxed and at ease.....

It's a warm, summer's day and the temperature is just right......all around you are green, mature trees, an array of beautiful wild flowers and fragrant scents.....you hear the sound of warm air rustling through the leaves on the trees.....and feel the soft, cool grass beneath your feet.....

In the distance you hear the sound of water from a shallow stream winding along your path.....as you move closer to the stream you notice stones at the bottom of the stream and see small fish darting about in the clear water.......the sound of the water and the beauty all around you....makes you feel so relaxed and calm.....

You feel so peaceful, calm and comfortable in this place......you find the perfect place to relax and laying a blanket down on the warm grass, you settle down onto the blanket, aware of the warmth of the sun.....

Closing your eyes.... you allow the wonderful warmth of the sun to relax and comfort your whole mind and body, moving down from the top of your head... to the very tips of your toes, bring relaxation, peace and a sense of wellbeing to your entire being....

Notice as the warmth spreads all around the muscles of your eyes and eyelids....relaxing and soothing everything in its path.....your cheeks, mouth and jaw muscles all begin to soften and relax.....as your tongue rests comfortably in your mouth.....notice as this lovely warmth, now spreads down through your neck and shoulders muscles......you feel completely relaxed, comfortable and at peace.....as the comforting warmth moves down the length of your spine....releasing all tension, as you allow yourself to let go and relax....

Now the warmth gently moves down your arms, hands and fingers, as they become soft, relaxed and comfortable.....you feel yourself starting to drift down into a feeling of deep relaxation and peace, as the warmth of the sun moves throughout your body.....you feel safe as you know that this beautiful garden (place) is a special place just for you.....

Now the warmth of the sun moves down the front of your body.....bringing relaxation to your chest, stomach and pelvis, soothing and comforting you and your baby with its warmth.....you breathe calmness and peace down to your baby.....tune into your baby now for a moment or two....letting them know that you can't wait to meet them and welcome them into the world...calmly and peacefully....

You feel confident and ready for the birth of your baby.....

The gentle warmth of the sun moves down your legs now, relaxing and softening the muscles of your legs, feet and toes.....as you move deeper and deeper into a sense of relaxation and at peace....your entire body is now bathed in soft, warm golden light....

And now as I count down from 10 to 1, with each number you progressively become more and more deeply relaxed and ease...

10...feeling deeply relaxed and at ease.... 9.... letting go of all tension....8....7, feeling calm .... 6...5.....drifting down and further down.....4.....it's so easy to let go and relax.....3 deeper and deeper relaxed.....2... and 1 feeling more relaxed than you can ever imagine.....

Enjoy this feeling of relaxation and peace for a moment or two now......this quality of relaxation and peace....that you have created in your body and mind......is available for you now, during your labour and birth and after your baby is born.....it allows your body to relax...soften...and open and do what it is designed to do...to give birth to your baby with ease....

Giving birth is a beautiful, natural and normal process....your body knows how to give birth to your baby.....growing and nurturing your baby perfectly.....as each day passes you become more and more confident and in tune with your body and your baby.....you instinctively trust your body to bring you to the start of labour at the right time for you, so that you bring your baby into the world calmly and comfortably.....

Every time you listen to this relaxation....you find that you relax more and more quickly, easily and deeply......your breathing is relaxed and calm...you feel calm, relaxed and well prepared for the birth of your baby....whatever turn your birth may take, you will welcome each surge with peace and calm confidence.....

Every time you focus on your relaxing breath, you feel calm and relaxed....this becomes second nature to you....an anchor of peace during your labour and birth...

As your labour progresses, with each surge, your relaxation and trust deepens.....each powerful, surge brings you closer and closer to meeting your baby.....you are strong and confident woman....taking everything, easily, in your stride, both now, during your baby's birth and after your baby born....

No matter what you are doing....you can always relax and connect with your breathing, slowing down your breath, focussing inwards....on your strength and power....

Every day you find the time to relax and nurture yourself by listening to this relaxation and connecting with your breathing practice.....enjoying the peace and confidence that it brings you.....

In a moment or two, it will be time for you to leave the garden and return to everyday reality....knowing that you can return to it any time that you want to....this sense of relaxation and peace is always available for you, whenever you need it...

And now I'm going to count from 1-5 and when I get to the number 5 you will be wide awake and alert, feeling relaxed, refreshed and ready to continue with your day....

If you would like to drift off into a restful, deep sleep, then this is absolutely fine....you will wake up feeling refreshed and relaxed...

1, beginning to become more aware of yourself now

2, feeling as if you are waking up from a pleasant doze

3, normal sensations returning to your fingers and toes

4, feeling more awake and alert

5, opening your eyes, feeling awake and aware, ready to continue with your day

Garden Relaxation – Birth Partner

This relaxation is for the birth partner to help them to feel calm, confident and ready to be the best support during labour & birth.

Again, when your partner reads this out to you feel free to replace the garden description below (in italics) with something else.

Just settle yourself into the most comfortable position and allow your eyes to gently close now......you don't have to stay absolutely still, but it may be that that's all you actually want to do......just to allow yourself to settle more and more deeply into the chair or on the bed....

Now take a deep breath in..... and let it out slowly......and allow yourself to become more relaxed as you do so......as though you are breathing away all tensions from your mind and body......

Now bring your attention to your breathing and allow your breathing to slow down and deepen....... as you breathe in, imagine calmness and relaxation going in....and as you breathe out each time, imagine tension drifting away from you.....

For a moment or two I wonder if you can imagine yourself walking in the most beautiful, peaceful garden.....a place where you feel completely comfortable, relaxed and at ease.....

It's a warm, summer's day and the temperature is just right......all around you are green, mature trees, an array of beautiful wild flowers and fragrant scents.....you hear the sound of warm air rustling through the leaves on the trees.....and feel the soft, cool grass beneath your feet.....

In the distance you hear the sound of water from a shallow stream winding along your path.....as you move closer to the stream you notice stones at the bottom of the stream and see small fish darting about in the clear water.......the sound of the water and the beauty all around you....makes you feel so relaxed and calm.....

You feel so peaceful, calm and comfortable in this place......you find the perfect place to relax and laying a blanket down on the warm grass, you settle down onto the blanket, aware of the warmth of the sun.....

Closing your eyes.... you allow the wonderful warmth of the sun to relax and comfort your whole mind and body, moving down from the top of your head... to the very tips of your toes, bring relaxation, peace and a sense of wellbeing to your entire being....

Notice as the warmth spreads all around the muscles of your eyes and eyelids....relaxing and soothing everything in its path.....your cheeks, mouth and jaw muscles all begin to soften and relax.....as your tongue rests comfortably in your mouth.....notice as this lovely warmth, now spreads down through your neck and shoulders muscles......you feel completely relaxed, comfortable and at peace.....as the comforting warmth moves down the length of your spine....releasing all tension, as you allow yourself to let go and relax....

Now the warmth gently moves down your arms, hands and fingers, as they become soft, relaxed and comfortable.....you feel yourself starting to drift down into a feeling of deep relaxation and peace, as the warmth of the sun moves throughout your body.....you feel safe as you know that this beautiful garden is a special place just for you.....

Now the warmth of the sun moves down the front of your body.....bringing relaxation to your chest, stomach and pelvis, soothing and comforting you with its warmth.....you breathe calmness and peace.....

You feel confident and ready to support your partner during the birth of your baby....

The gentle warmth of the sun moves down your legs now, relaxing and softening the muscles of your legs, feet and toes.....as you move deeper and deeper into a sense of relaxation and at peace....your entire body is now bathed in soft, warm golden light....

And now as I count down from 10 to 1, with each number you progressively become more and more deeply relaxed and ease...

10...feeling deeply relaxed and at ease.... 9.... letting go of all tension....8....7, feeling calm .... 6...5.....drifting down and further down.....4.....it's so easy to let go and relax.....3 deeper and deeper relaxed.....2... and 1 feeling more relaxed than you can ever imagine.....

Enjoy this feeling of relaxation and peace for a moment or two now......this quality of relaxation and peace....that you have created in your body and mind......is available for you now, during your baby's birth and after your baby is born.....it allows your body to relax...your breathing to be calm and your mind clear, focused and knowing exactly how best to support your partner during labour....

Giving birth is a beautiful, natural and normal process....your partner's body knows how to do this perfectly.... each time you carry out your practice together you feel more and more confident and in tune with her and her needs and wishes at this exciting time in both your lives. You instinctively trust your intuition to know how to support her through each stage of your baby's birth so she is able to bring your baby into the world calmly and comfortably, with you strong and supportive every step of the way.

Every time you listen to this relaxation....you find that you relax more and more quickly, easily and deeply......your breathing is relaxed and calm...you feel well prepared for the birth of your baby....whatever turn the birth may take, you will know exactly what to do to best support your partner with unwavering strength, energy and confidence.....

Every time you focus on your relaxing breath, you feel calm and relaxed....this becomes second nature to you....an anchor of peace and confidence during the labour and birth...

As the labour progresses, with every surge you trust that you know what to do and you take everything, easily, in your stride....

No matter what may be going on in the birth room you can always relax and connect with your breathing, slowing down your breath, focussing inwards....on your strength and in turn, sending this strength to your partner leaving her feeling fully supported and able to let go into the birthing process, knowing you are there for her every step of the way.

Every day you find the time to relax yourself by listening to this relaxation and connecting with your breathing practice.....enjoying the peace and confidence that it brings you.....

In a moment or two, it will be time for you to leave the garden and return to everyday reality….knowing that you can return to it any time that you want to….this sense of relaxation, confidence and peace is always available for you, whenever you need it…

And now I'm going to count from 1-5 and when I get to the number 5 you will be wide awake and alert, feeling relaxed, refreshed and ready to continue with your day….

If you would like to drift off into a restful, deep sleep, then this is absolutely fine….you will wake up feeling refreshed and relaxed…

1, beginning to become more aware of yourself now

2, feeling as if you are waking up from a pleasant dose

3, normal sensations returning to your fingers and toes

4, feeling more awake and alert

5, opening your eyes, feeling awake and aware, ready to continue with your day

Baby Bumps' Positive Birth Stories

Below are a few positive birth stories for different birth scenarios. All are from clients, with their names removed for confidentiality. These birth stories, and others, are shared with permission on my website.

Home birth:

"Hi Jackie,

I am sitting with my beautiful little 4 week old baby daughter sleeping beside me and thought I would take this opportunity to write to you to say a huge thank you. We had such a wonderful birthing experience and couldn't have done it without the tools you provided us with during our Hypnobirthing course. I gave birth in the water, at home and with no pain relief. The birth we had both wished for!

My first surge was a 6.30pm and actually took place while listening to a hypnobirthing track! My husband came home from work an hour or so later, at which point I was having a surge every 20 minutes or so. He set up a mattress in the living room with candles and calm music. He talked me through every surge, encouraging me to breathe and relax as we had practiced. I used a tens machine which really helped. He called the midwife at about 2am when the surges were longer and more frequent, and by the time she arrived I was 7cm dilated. The pool was now ready in our dining room (it took a long time to fill!) and my husband had used our fairy lights and music to create the same calm atmosphere. I was anxious about removing the tens machine but the warm water felt wonderful.

Again, my husband was a huge support, physically and emotionally. Although I found it challenging to relax as I had

174

done when we'd practiced, I was certainly more relaxed than I would have been without our hypnobirthing mindsets. The music really helped as I associated this with the relaxation sessions I had been doing for the past few weeks.

For the next few hours my waters were being a bit stubborn and I decided to have them broken, after which things moved fairly quickly.

Our little girl was born at 9am and it was by far the best moment of our lives. I held her for 20 minutes in the water before my husband cut the cord and had some skin to skin time with her himself. The midwife stayed with us until lunch time to make sure we were happy with feeding and left us snuggled up as a family to get to know our little baby girl. Four weeks later she still hasn't been to a hospital!

I would recommend hypnobirthing and if possible home birth so highly. You played such a significant part in our journey to our dream birth. THANK YOU!

Second time mother:

Hi Jackie,

So sorry for not getting back to you sooner!!!!

All is well here thanks, baby 'L' is gorgeous, and 'P' is enjoying having a baby to play with!

The birth was very different to 'P's'... I managed to get through most of the contractions at home by breathing and focusing on music, as practised. Eventually she was born 20mins after I was measured being at 4cm dilated!! We didn't even make it to the labour ward! But I feel happy and pleased with how things went, and proud of how I coped – only having gas & air!

Thanks for all your help and support in the preparation.

Second time mother who was induced:

Hi Jackie

I thought I'd email to let you know that I gave birth to my daughter last Wednesday, and the hypnobirthing techniques were very successful.

In the end I had to be induced at 40+12. I was warned that the pessary could cause pain, and to expect it to take at least 24 hours, so even though I started having contractions after a few hours, I was managing it so well with the breathing and visualisations that I didn't realise that I was actually in labour. As the contractions intensified I was so 'in the zone' that none of the staff realised I was in labour either, until my waters suddenly broke. Unfortunately with all the fussing about what to do with me as the birthing centre and labour ward were full, not to mention a very intense and fast labour, I lost the flow in the final stage, so it wasn't a super calm birth, but it wasn't a nightmare ordeal like my first one and I didn't need any pain relief apart from my TENS machine and gas and air. After my waters broke it only took about an hour until my daughter was born – I didn't even leave the antenatal ward, though they did manage to wheel me into a private room at the last minute so I didn't have to give birth in a corridor.

Incidentally, I think that one of the most useful things in the course for me was when you demonstrated to us how time passes much more quickly when you take slow breaths, in that exercise where we counted how many breaths we took in one minute, or something similar – knowing that to be the case, it really helped make the contractions more bearable in early labour.

So, thank you for your help, the course and materials were clearly very effective and worthwhile

Second time mother whose baby arrived early:

Hi Jackie. I have been meaning to email you,

He came 3 weeks early and oh my did the hypnobirthing help! I think it really preserved my energy for when I needed it, I also think the midwives underestimated my progress as I was so silent. My actual labour was about an hour!

Not just the birth but also think it helped with me calming down as an individual. I started to cramp and saw my mucus plug 3 weeks early but still managed to present to the CEO, go Boots and M&S to get baby bits, pack up my desk and go home to pack, all done with whilst calm, happy and no panic at all!

Thank you so much, I'm a very, very happy mum and really enjoyed the newborn phase this time round.

Also thanks for empowering me to take off and throw away the belts they put around you which totally restricted my thoughts and movements!*

*during a course we talk about requesting intermittent monitoring, if appropriate

First time mother who had an assisted birth:

Hi Jackie

What a week!!

As you know my waters broke last Tuesday and then my contractions began around 6pm on the Wednesday evening- I went into hospital and was already 5cms dilated! Unfortunately I had to stay on labour ward rather than go to the birthing centre as my waters had gone over 24hrs previous so the baby had to be monitored throughout. I laboured without any pain relief and just used the breathing techniques we had learned until 6.30am on Thursday when it became apparent baby was unable to make her way out alone! Baby was born with the help of a kiwi cap (and a spinal block!) at 7.53am 30th April!!

All of the staff commented on the relaxed nature of the labour and how I coped with the contractions and baby was born with fantastic apgar scores despite the long labour. 'A' helped massively during the more intense contractions by reading out some of the scripts we had practised and it really focused me.

Thank you for all of your help and support it was so appreciated. Although we had to deviate from our birth plan I believe the Hypnobirthing techniques we used were hugely beneficial when it came to making important decisions about the direction of the birth."

First time mother who had a fast active labour:

"Hi Jackie,

'R' is doing really well. It's so surreal being parents, we're loving it despite total sleep deprivation.

My active labour ended up being 1 hour 25 minutes and I had her in the pool at the birth centre – only just. She came out in her sac so her head appeared like a little astronaut. She was 10 days overdue and was 7 pounds 3 oz and it was a totally natural birth.

I had contractions from 1am at home, was in hospital at 4.30 and told I was 1 cm. My contractions were regular and 3/4 a minute from the get go so they told us to go for a walk for an hour. When I went back at about 6am, I was still one centimetre dilated, so was sent across to the labour ward. Things must have progressed rapidly there, because pretty soon I was feeling an incredibly strong urge to push. A midwife measured me and said I was fully dilated and ready to push, so they whizzed me back to the birth unit, where I had to get into the pool straight away. Two pushes later she was born.

R was brilliant reminding me of the breathing techniques and remaining calm when the surges were at their most intense. The visualisations kept me very focused and confirmed to me the power of the mind body connection. We were the talk of the birth unit as to how quickly everything happened.

So delighted to have had such a positive experience and he is such content little baby. Thanks so much Jackie."

First time mother – waterbirth

Dear Jackie,

We are writing to thank you for the invaluable information you provided to us in the hypnobirthing course we attended in December.

Our son, was born on February 1st weighing 7lb 8oz in the XXX midwife led unit. The techniques you taught us for breathing and relaxation along with the use of water and counter pressure all allowed me to stick to our birth plan and have a drug free delivery. I definitely couldn't have done it without P's support and hypnobirthing had absolutely prepared him for every stage of the labour- he was my advocate, cheerleader and guide throughout.

Thank you for arming us with the information we needed to make choices that helped us bring our son safely and naturally into the world. Attached is a picture of our sweet boy just hours after his birth and a family shot taken earlier this week.

Thank you again X

First time mother and informed decision making

Jackie, better late than never, my birth story:

'S' was born 13 days late. From day 1 post my due date inductions were proposed to me. I declined to have a sweep at day 1 past my due date but after a week I did have a sweep as I had been experiencing Braxton Hicks and also on examination I had begun to dilate, therefore things were already on the move. I had a 2nd sweep at 10 days past my due date and at 12 days past D Day went to discuss my options with a consultant.

The consultant examined me and I was 2.5 cm dilated by this point and I could feel 'S' was much lower down, I was also experiencing stronger Braxton Hicks. Incidentally they found my fluid levels were slightly low and so the doctor advised I was admitted there and then to have my waters broken in theatre. I sought a 2nd opinion about this and spoke with 2 senior midwives, I was advised that my fluid levels could have been low for a while and they weren't dangerously low.

I went against the doctor's advice, this was quite scary as I had to sign a consent form to self discharge. I went into labour naturally that night and gave birth naturally to 'S' in the midwife led unit. I used the birthing pool and shower along with relaxation techniques and breathing control throughout the 2nd stage of labour.

Hypnobirthing gave me the confidence and the knowledge to question the health professionals' advice & plans to induce me. I'm so glad I did as I managed a natural birth, and during monitoring 'S''s heart rate was always normal so I feel that she entered the world in the best way possible and was not distressed"

First time mother:

Hey Jackie!

Been meaning to email you! Well basically my waters went on Thursday as I was walking up the stairs in the hospital to go have a blood pressure check! I wasn't having contractions so they booked me in for an induction the next morning.

So I went home and walked loads went and had labour reflexology and then thought I best just sleep! The next morning I was having gentle period like cramps but they told me to come in anyway. I went in and at about 10.30am they put me in the induction ward.

The midwife came to give me the pessary and then said she couldn't as I was already 3cm. I said to her I was getting period pains so she decided to leave me to it for a while.

Anyway out of nowhere it felt like they went from period pains to full on contractions. They seemed to last minimum 90 seconds and then the gap between them was getting shorter and shorter.

I wasn't being checked on as I think as a first time mum they thought I'd be there for ages. Suddenly there was no let up between contractions and I thought if that wasn't transition I really needed drugs!! (I did have gas and air but made me feel sick I couldn't use it) so I literally screamed the place down for a midwife — she came and examined me and I was 9cm.

I just knew I had to get out of the ward and into a delivery room' (poor people who were in there with me! I think I panicked as nobody was around to check on me hence the screaming for a midwife!)

I am laughing now because they kept on about being high risk and constant monitoring!

So anyway at 5.35pm our little boy made an appearance! He weighed 6pound 2 oz was 53cm long. Midwives in delivery suite were amazing! I think I'd lost the plot by time I got into the delivery suite and was being a bit of a nightmare then! But once I got in I didn't panic at all during the pushing stage even when he got a little stuck and it took a bit longer – I think all the hypnobirthing helped with that – no tears or episiotomy thank goodness!

Funny thing is I so wanted to be able to move around and all I could do to get comfortable was lie down in the end!! I tried kneeling and standing for birth but I found lying down the best!

Funny how you think one thing but another thing actually happens!

Glad to be home and working out a newborn! He's so cute! Thanks for all your help and advice it definitely worked! Xxx

First time mother with short hospital time:

Hi Jackie

We had our baby on Saturday 21 February at 5.39 pm and weighing in at 7 lb 5 oz and with no complications. He arrived one day before his due date.

We think the hypnobirthing really helped us. I started having mild contractions around 8pm on the Friday night but I managed to sleep through parts of the night, we spent the morning and early afternoon at home as the contractions had not reached a regular pattern, but by early afternoon they started getting quicker albeit I would have a couple of contractions 2-3 minutes apart and then might have a gap of 8-10 minutes and they were varying in length from 30 seconds to around a minute. By the time we reached the hospital at 4 pm I was 7-8 cm dilated. We had half an hour on the labour ward (for an unknown reason the birth centre was closed) using some gas and air, by which point I was fully dilated and baby was born naturally 40 minutes later.

We credit the short time in hospital to the preparation we did with the hypnobirthing. Thank you for your assistance.

Further reading
Mullen, J. 'Hypnobirthing the art to a peaceful birth', RCM, 2012. Available at: https://www.rcm.org.uk/news-views-andanalysis/
analysis/hypnobirthing-the-art-to-a-peaceful-birth

Baker, K. 'On Focus. How To Support Hypnobirthing', *Midwives,* Issue 5, 2014. Available at
https://www.rcm.org.uk/sites/default/files/34-35_0.pdf

http://www.royhunter.com/hypnotherapy-faq.htm

I'M EXPECTING A BABY

15

PAIN MANAGEMENT OPTIONS

When it comes to pain management of course there is no 'one size fits all', and while some women are very focused on utilising the incredible tools they already have within themselves, others may have this in mind, but also want to explore medical options - or their initial preferences change during their labour.

In this chapter we will look at the options available, so you are able to make an informed decision when the time comes. Some methods have already been covered but a recap is offered in this chapter.

Hypnobirthing

To recap the previous chapter, hypnobirthing is a popular and effective method that uses deep relaxation, breathing, visualisations, mindset overhaul and fear-release techniques to manage labour. Birth partners are very much involved from the outset and have a clear role in assisting their partner. Time is spent before the birth practising the techniques and working on releasing fear.

Pros

- Women and partners feel empowered.

- Birth partners are very much involved.

- Often no medication is needed.

- Women are informed and educated about how their body works in labour.

- Women report feeling calm and in control whatever turn their birth takes.

- No side effects for mother or baby – babies benefit from the increased oxygen from the constant deep breathing.

Cons

- There is a cost to do a course or to buy any book/s and MP3s.

- You need to practise in advance (which is lovely!).

- Some women find it only gets them to a certain point in their labour.

Breathing techniques

I know we've talked about this a lot already, but it cannot be underestimated! Deep, slow breathing is calming and brings valuable oxygen and a good blood flow to both mother and baby. Partners can be involved and can assist by using co-breathing if the mother starts to become panicked. Relaxed breathing has many benefits and will be a woman's best friend in labour – whatever other choices she may make.

Pros

- It is free!

- It increases blood and oxygen flow to mother and baby.

- Birth partners can be involved.

- It instantly reduces stress and tension.

- It gives a woman great focus.

- It increases birth hormones like oxytocin and endorphins, which help a woman feel calm and relaxed and her make her surges more efficient.

- No side effects for mother or baby; both will benefit from relaxed breathing.

Cons

- It takes time and effort to practise the breathing (which is well worth it!).

- Some women find breathing techniques only get them so far before they want additional methods.

Massage

Touch is comforting for most, although some women prefer not to be touched during labour. Touch can vary and includes gentle stroking, holding, firmer stroking, foot massage, hand massage and deep massage using palms or knuckles and counter-pressure. Usually the firmer massage is welcomed in the latter stages of labour. Touch may help a woman feel safe and secure and increases the production of the hormone oxytocin. It is a way for a partner to communicate with the woman, letting her know they are there for her without using words.

You can use certain essential oils diluted in a carrier oil, as mentioned earlier.

Pros

- Provides comfort.

- Increases oxytocin and endorphin production.

- Birth partners are involved.

- No side effects for mother or baby.

Cons

- Some women do not want to be touched in labour.

- Some women want additional methods.

Active birth (positions and movement)

Active birth is when a woman follows her body's lead and moves accordingly, rather than being tethered to the bed, on her back, which makes contractions slower and more uncomfortable.

There are numerous studies on the benefits of using positions and The Royal College of Obstetricians & Gynaecologists (RCOG) recommends that women be encouraged to assume whatever position is most comfortable for them.

When a woman is supine (on her back), blood supply to the uterus and placenta is restricted due to the weight of the uterus pressing on certain blood vessels. Her blood pressure can also drop in this position. Being upright increases the pelvic outlet by up to a third, helping the baby move down as well as making the mother feel more comfortable.

Pros

- Movement and changing position are a good distraction and provide a focus.

- When you follow your instinctive urge to move it may encourage your baby into a good position and will makes things feel more manageable.

- UFO positions create more room in the pelvis for the baby.

Cons

- You may feel tired, in which case you can lie on your left side to rest for a while.

Continuous support

There is much evidence which points to the benefits of a woman having a familiar, constant and calming birth partner present. This is why a home birth can be such a great option, as you may well have met your midwife several times in advance of the birth.

Emotional support boosts you and helps you feel supported and confident. Some women or couples decide to hire a doula for this very reason and doulas have been shown to reduce the need for pharmacological pain relief.

If your birth partner is someone who is likely to panic or is concerned about how best they can support you, hiring a doula or having a second birth partner available will be beneficial. When someone is nervous or frightened they will be pumping out adrenalin into the room making it harder for you to relax and go within.

Water birth

Many women use water during their labour, and this can include getting into a shower, a bath or a specially designed birth pool, which is either plumbed in or inflated. If you are planning a home birth you will need to make arrangements to hire or buy one. Some home birth teams have these available for hire.

The soothing effects of water work best when you are around halfway through your labour, at roughly 5cm dilated. You can have all of your labour in the pool, or part of it. Some women prefer to have the second stage out of the pool, but it's entirely your choice.

Most midwives prefer that a woman has the third stage (delivery of the placenta) out of the pool in case she feels faint, and it is easier to assess blood loss when not in the water.

Research shows that women who use water in labour are less likely to use pain medication.

Pros

- Enhances a feeling of privacy as you are immersed in the pool/bath.

- The buoyancy of the water allows for greater ease of movement.

- You can use gas and air in the pool.

- If you don't like it you can just get out.

Cons

- It may not be available when you go into labour.

- It cannot be used if you need to be closely monitored or if you have had recent opioids (pain-relieving drugs).

- If a problem is suspected for you or your baby you will be asked to get out.

- If you find your labour slows whilst in the water you may like to get out, walk about and then get back in later. In fact it is good practice to get out every few hours and walk around a bit.

Gas and air (Entonox)

Gas and air is a mix of 50 per cent oxygen and 50 per cent nitrous oxide. In the UK it is available at home births and also in all birth centre and hospital settings. You inhale the gas through a mouthpiece. It takes the edge off the surges and can make you feel a bit giggly and light-headed.

Pros

- It can encourage deep breathing and increased oxygen flow.

- It is readily available everywhere (in the UK).

- It is short lasting so if you do not like the effects once you stop using it they wear off quickly.

- It won't hinder your birth or cause problems for your baby and the increased oxygen may be beneficial.

- You won't need any additional monitoring while using it.

- You are in control of how and when you use it.

- You can still move around while using it.

- You can use it in the birth pool.

Cons

- The effects are mild – but this may be all you need!

- While you can still move, you will be a bit restricted due to holding onto the mouthpiece.

- Some women feel drowsy or nauseous and some are sick.

- It can dry your mouth out, so have regular sips of water and apply lip balm to help with this.

- It can take a bit of getting used to in order to get the timing right, so it is most effective at the peak of the surge (take a couple of deep breaths of the gas and air at the very start of the surge to maximise the effects and this should see you through that surge).

TENS machine (Transcutaneous Electrical Nerve Stimulation)

A TENS machine for labour is a small handheld device with four sticky pads, which you attach to your skin on either side of your spine. It can be clipped on to your clothing if you prefer not to hold it. It delivers safe electrical pulses of current through the wires/pads, which give a tingly sensation.

Usually a woman starts on the lowest level and works her way up by turning the dial bit by bit as her labour progresses. Some machines have a boost button which can be pressed at the peak of a surge, but remember to turn this off afterwards so you feel the benefit next time.

There is not much evidence available on the effectiveness of TENS machines, nor is it known exactly how they work. It is likely that they work by a combination of the following:

- The electrical pulses you receive muddle the pain message the brain receives.

- The tingly sensation stimulates endorphin production, the body's natural and powerful painkiller.

- They give a feeling of control and offer distraction.

Usually hospitals and birth centres do not provide TENS machines, so it is up to you to hire or buy one. Not all TENS machines are suitable for labour, so make sure you hire or buy one that is appropriate.

It is best to set up the TENS machine when you are in early labour rather than established labour when your surges are strong. It can take a while for it to take effect, so try it for a hour or so before you decide whether or not it is working for you.

Pros

- A TENS machine will not affect your labour or your baby.

- Other options will still be open to you (apart from a water birth (unless you remove the pads/machine!).

- If you do not like the sensation you can just turn the machine off and remove the pads.

- It can provide distraction and a feeling of control.

- You can move freely.

- You purchase a TENS machine, or hire or borrow one, and can set it up yourself (your birth partner will need to stick the pads in the right place on your back) without the need for a midwife or doctor.

Cons

- The pads can lose their stickiness, but a drop of water on them can help if this happens, or you can buy some spares.

- You cannot use the birth pool/shower/bath with the machine on.

- Your partner will not be able to massage your lower back.

- Do not use a TENS machine if you have a pacemaker, before you are in labour, before 37 weeks unless under medical supervision, or if you have epilepsy.

- If you do decide to try one, pack spare batteries!

- Some women say they find using a TENS machine means they are waiting for the next surge so they can press buttons, rather than staying in their zone.

Opioids such as pethidine & diamorphine

Opiate/opioid painkillers are medicines with effects similar to morphine. They are usually given as an injection in the thigh and, as it can often make a woman feel sick, an anti-sickness drug is normally given at the same time which isn't always effective.

Opioids can be given in differing doses. If you are very sensitive to drugs or are of a slight build, you may want to ask about starting on a lower dose.

Pros

- Some women find opioids help them relax and get some sleep particularly if they have had a long first stage of labour and they are shattered or highly stressed.

- A midwife can administer pethidine and sometimes diamorphine so there is no need to wait for a doctor should you want this.

- It produces a sedation effect that can be helpful for some women who may be feeling very anxious.

- If you are in established labour it appears not to slow things down.

- It may postpone or prevent a woman from having an epidural if this is something she would prefer to avoid for reasons personal to her.

Cons

- Some people do not like the effects of opioids and it takes several hours for the effects to wear off.

- Women may feel some of these sensations: euphoric, dizzy, drowsy, spaced out, detached and sedated - making labour harder to cope with.

- Opioids can make some women feel sick and vomit despite the anti-sickness drug.

- All opioids cross the placenta and on occasion the baby may be slower to initiate breathing straight after birth. This is why opiods are not given in the later stages of labour.

- Opioids may make getting feeding your baby off to a good start difficult.

- If the drug is given close to the baby's birth it will take the baby several days to work it out of her system.

- Opioids only provide limited pain relief.

- It is likely that you will not be able to use the birth pool until the effects have worn off, however timings around this vary from Trust to Trust.

Epidural

Epidural analgesia is around 90 per cent effective in removing all pain and most of the feeling from around the waist down. It is a local anaesthetic injected into the epidural space between the vertebrae of the back and requires an anaesthetist to set it up.

You will be given a local anaesthetic in your back so you won't feel the epidural being inserted, though you will feel some pressure as this takes place. Occasionally it may not work and will need to be adjusted or taken out and reinserted.

An anaesthetist may not be available right away and you may have to wait for them. It takes around 20 minutes to insert an epidural and 20 minutes for it to take its full effect, which may be worth bearing in mind.

Pros

- It gives total pain relief in most cases.

- Once it is set up it does not require an anaesthetist to top it up – a midwife can do this or the woman can self administer a top up via an epidural pump if this option is available.

- Some women are able to sleep and rest for a while as there is no (or very little) sensation felt, even though you may be aware of your contractions.

Cons

- Around 10 per cent of women only experience partial pain relief.

- You need to be on the labour ward to have an epidural.

- You need to be able to hold still when it is being set up and if you are not able to do so, the anaesthetist may decide it is not safe for them to go ahead.

- The sensations of birth encourage a woman to move about, which helps her baby get into a good position. With an epidural you will not be able to move around freely, which may slow your labour down.

- It takes about 40 minutes before you feel the effects.

- There is an increased chance of a needing forceps or suction (ventouse) birth. Having an epidural will mean continuous monitoring of the baby's heart rate and careful monitoring of the mother.

- You may not have normal sensation when you need to wee so a catheter might need to be inserted to empty the bladder.

- You may need to be given drugs to augment your labour.

- There is a chance of lowered blood pressure, therefore you need an intravenous infusion (drip) to ensure a safe epidural procedure. This drip may be used for other reasons, such as to give medication to speed your labour up or if you are being sick.

- The baby needs to be monitored closely using electronic foetal monitoring. This type of monitoring is associated with a higher rate of surgical delivery.

- Usually a woman will be lying down after an epidural, so the powerful effects of gravity are not utilised. You can ask your midwife for help with moving onto your side or sitting more upright if you wish to – some hospital beds can be positioned in an upright chair position. Ask if there is a peanut ball to help with opening of the pelvis. A peanut ball is a birth ball shaped like a monkey nut and it can be positioned between the woman's legs to help with opening.

- Second stage will be longer and you are more likely to require synthetic oxytocin to speed this up.

- You may feel itchy.

- You may develop a fever as raised temperature is associated with an epidural. A raised temperature can cause staff to consider the possibility of infection, which then leads to increased monitoring and the offer of treatment with antibiotics.

- Some women experience a severe headache that can last for days or weeks if not treated. If you develop a headache talk to your midwife or anaesthetist.

- A low-dose epidural (so-called 'mobile epidurals', even though you won't be fully mobile, just less heavy legged) may mean in the early hours you will be able to move about with help but the more top-ups you have the more heavy-legged you will feel and the less likely you are able to move freely.

Further reading

http://www.labourpains.com/ui/content/content.aspx?id=45

OAA (Obstetrics Anaesthetists Association)
http://mobile.oaaformothers.info/

http://www.which.co.uk/birth-choice/faqs

https://evidencebasedbirth.com covers many pain relief
options in detail including breathing, relaxation, epidurals,
waterbirth, etc.

16

DUE DATES AND INDUCTION

It is easy and understandable to become fixated on the so-called 'due date' you have been given to predict your baby's arrival. Based on best evidence, there is no such thing as an exact due date and the estimated due date of 40 weeks is not accurate, with only around 4–5 per cent of babies arriving at this time.

Initially your midwife will ask you the date of the first day of your last period. For women with an average length cycle (28 days) that date is considered to be about two weeks before conception. She will then add on 40 weeks from the first day of your last period to generate a due date. Then at the 12 week ultrasound scan, measurements of the baby are taken and the due date may change to take these into account.

The problem is being fixated on pregnancy lasting 40 weeks as for many women this is not the case and it is odd that we assume all babies take exactly the same time to gestate and be ready to be born!

Most babies are born between 38 and 42 weeks of pregnancy (often called 'at term'). So even if you are sure of your conception date, birth can vary up to around 4 weeks.

For a healthy mother who has no other factors to consider, being born 'late' rarely causes problems for the baby. However, after 42 weeks there is a small but statistically significant increase in risk, though there is no exact time, as in everything becomes risk laden the moment she hits 42+1. Incredibly sadly, stillbirth can happen at any gestation. Since there is a small increase in risk past 42 weeks, induction of labour, which is starting labour off artificially using drugs, is usually offered between 41+0 and 42+0 weeks. This varies though with some healthcare professionals offering induction of labour at 41 weeks to take into account that sometimes the induction process and birth takes a few days, so best to start before 42 weeks.

Placenta 'failure' late in pregnancy

Dr Sara Wickham is a midwife, educator, author and researcher who has written many books, and recently updated her book '*Inducing Labour – making informed decisions*' which is highly recommended if you are being offered induction of labour and want to know the research and evidence on it all.

In her book Dr Wickham talks about there being no evidence that placenta insufficiency happens at a particular time in pregnancy, or at the same time for all women and babies. She also says that "there is no doubt that a few women will have problems with their placentas, but this can occur at any time at (say) 15 weeks, 23 weeks or 32 weeks of pregnancy"

I often hear the words 'they won't let me go past 'X' weeks and are going to induce me'. But the choice to accept or decline induction of labour is yours. If a woman declines she will be offered additional checks, such as monitoring every 2–3 days when past 42 weeks and an additional ultrasound scan to monitor the depth of the pool of liquor (waters) around the baby — an indication of how the placenta is functioning. You will be invited into hospital to have your baby's heartbeat listened to electronically. As ever, it is important to keep monitoring your baby's movements during this time and to get checked out if there is any change in this.

What starts labour?

It is not known exactly how labour starts. Consider your due date as estimate rather than something that is set in stone — think of your baby being due in the first or second half of a particular month.

In the last few days of pregnancy some women feel great, while others feel like they have had enough. It can be helpful to remember all the amazing things you and your baby are doing behind the scenes to prepare for the onset of labour.

- Your baby is putting the last finishing touches to the development of his lungs.

- In the third trimester your baby's brain grows faster than ever.

- He is growing more so called 'brown fat' which will keep him warm once he arrives.

- Your uterus is growing more oxytocin receptors, priming it for your baby's birth.

- You are passing valuable antibodies to your baby.

How does induction of labour work?

Induction of labour is when your labour is started artificially, using medical methods. There is a non-medical method called a 'membrane sweep', an internal examination which your midwife can do to try to encourage labour to start.

Why might a woman be offered induction of labour?

- Your midwife or obstetrician may feel that factors such as age, weight or health issues mean it is safer to have your labour induced. If this is the case, you can ask for more specific research and information on this - such as statistics for your particular situation - so you are able to make an informed decision.

- Your waters may have released but labour has not started. If your waters release and labour has not started after 1–2 days, this may slightly increase the chance of infection, so induction of labour is offered. Ask what is the relative risk of 'X, Y or X' is versus the absolute risk. For example the relative risk of 'X' may be that the risk doubles, but the absolute risk may be that that risk goes from 1%-2% - the latter being a far less scary picture.

- Your baby may be considered to be 'overdue' (the most common reason for induction is prolonged pregnancy). But are they really overdue? Some women may have very short, long or erratic menstrual cycles and ovulation can occur at different times during a cycle. Discuss your specific situation with a senior midwife if you feel you're unsure about the due date you've been given.

- Reduced movements. A baby's movements should not slow down.

- The baby's growth rate may be in question. But NICE do not currently recommend induction of labour if a health care professional suspects a baby is larger than expected for gestational age (unless there are other factors in place). Dating and growth scans are not 100% accurate with many women being told they are having very large babies or very small babies whose babies are born around a perfectly average weight!

Why might you decline induction of labour?

- You may prefer to wait for your baby to arrive when he is ready.

- You may feel well and be feeling your baby move regularly and consistently.

- You may feel the reason induction is being offered is not clinically justified.

There are a few different methods of trying to induce your labour; they are usually offered in the order in which they are discussed below.

Membrane sweep, or 'stretch and sweep'

In some hospitals a membrane sweep is offered at 40 weeks for a first-time mother and 41 weeks for subsequent babies, and can be carried out by a midwife or doctor. Membranes are the sac that encases your baby and the amniotic fluid.

If you consent to this procedure, the midwife or doctor will sweep or circle their finger around and inside your cervix. If the cervix is closed the midwife cannot perform a sweep.

A sweep may or may not encourage your body to go into labour. Sweeps are not recommended if your waters have released and labour has not yet started, as this may increase the risk of infection.

Sweeps can be repeated over several days if you wish. Many women find a membrane sweep uncomfortable and they can cause cramping and bleeding. Sometimes a sweep may inadvertently break a woman's waters, that which has its own set of risks including increased pain and an increase in the chance of infection.

As with all interventions offered, it's up to you whether you accept or decline a sweep. You can see if labour starts naturally, or decline a sweep at 40 weeks but request one at a later date.

Induction of Labour

This is a package that comprises of three parts, prostaglandins, artificial rupture of membranes (breaking a woman's waters) and intravenous syntocinon (synthetic oxytocin) and with it comes the need for regular internal examinations, to see how the cervix is responding (or not) to the drugs given.

Prostaglandin

Prostaglandin is a hormone that helps to soften the cervix and may help start labour by mimicking the natural prostaglandins that do this in preparation for labour. It is inserted into the woman's vagina, behind the cervix. It looks like a pessary or it can be a gel or sometimes like a small tampon ('propess'). There are several possible side effects some of these are hyperstimulation of the uterus, a headache, an irregular heartbeat and feeling sick.

Midwives can administer prostaglandins on the antenatal ward. They will monitor your baby's heart before and after the procedure. After it has been inserted you will need to rest for around 30 – 60 minutes to allow it to start being absorbed, and then you can move about or go for a walk.

With the propess used for induction of labour after careful monitoring, it may be suggested that you go home for 24 hours, or until contractions start if that is sooner, but not all hospitals offer this as an option.

Prostaglandins may cause period like contractions and sometimes cause the woman to have a bit of an upset stomach.

The process can be repeated again if it does not work, or a caesarean birth may be offered if your doctor feels this it may be a safer for you and your baby. You can talk through the reasons for recommending a caesarean and make sure you fully understand why this is being recommended and agree to it.

Sometimes prostaglandins can cause very fast, strong and intense contractions (hyperstimulation), which may cause problems for your baby. This is why induction of labour is performed in hospital. If this happens your midwife or doctor will remove the propess if this is what you have had, and/or give you drugs to stop this.

Artificial Rupture of Membranes (ARM) – also known as 'breaking the waters'

This procedure can be carried out by the midwife or doctor and is part of the induction process. It is also sometimes offered to speed up a slow labour (augmentation).

What is the process of ARM?

Your midwife or doctor will make a small break in the membranes surrounding your baby by using a special long, thin hook. It is worth asking if there is the option to wait a while after your waters have been broken as sometimes this alone can set labour off. Is it possible you could go for a walk, be gently active then rest on your own for a bit before moving on to the next step which follows ARM?

IVI Syntocinon (Pitocin in the USA)

Syntocinon is an artificial version of the hormone oxytocin. It is part of the induction of labour process and is set up after ARM if contractions have not become established, with dilation of the cervix. Syntocinon is given through an intravenous drip, which causes more regular contractions to establish (ARM also causes contractions). As syntocinon can sometimes cause over-stimulation of the uterus your baby's heart rate will need to be monitored continuously to check that it is within normal limits. Syntocinon is easily adjusted if a problem occurs.

Syntocinon has quite a few side effects, similar to prostaglandins, one of which is that it does not allow for a slow build-up of labour contractions and endorphins and is likely to be more intense and challenging than a natural labour, so an epidural is offered. Some women accept this, while others prefer to see how they go and use breathing, gas and air and/or hypnobirthing techniques.

Induction of labour increases the chance of having an assisted delivery using forceps or ventouse, which you can read about in the relevant chapter. It also increases the chances of needing a caesarean birth.

Other side effects of induction of labour

According to NICE, when labour was started using drugs:

- less than two-thirds of these women gave birth without further intervention with there being an increased

chance of a woman needing a
birth (such as forceps or vent
chance in a woman having a ca

Induction of labour has a large impact
and their babies and so needs to be cl

What if induction doesn't work?

You will have a discussion with your obstetrician. They may suggest another dose of prostaglandins or a caesarean birth may be offered in some circumstances.

Questions you can ask prior to accepting induction of labour

- What is the reason I am being offered induction?

- What are the benefits of induction of labour for my specific situation?

- What are the risks (to me or my baby), and how likely are they?

- What pain relief is available and when can I have it?

- What happens if I decline induction of labour?

- If I am booked in for induction and the labour ward fills up with women going into spontaneous labour, what will happen to my appointment? If it will be shifted back this may give you more of an idea how crucial (or not) a particular date is.

e professionals offering induction of labour

- Allow the woman time to discuss the information with her partner before coming to a decision.

- Encourage the woman to look at a variety of sources of information.

- Invite the woman to ask questions, and encourage her to think about her options.

- Support the woman in whatever decision she makes (NICE)

When guidelines are written, they are based on the whole nation rather than your specific situation. You should be given personalised information about the benefits and risks for you and your baby, as well as any alternatives.

If you feel unsure about whether or not you want to accept induction of labour or you don't feel you are being given personalised information, you can request to go through your notes and health background with a senior midwife, consultant midwife or Professional Maternity Advocate (PMA) and make a personalised plan. To make contact with any of the above just call your main hospital number and ask to be put through to one of them and perhaps ask for an email address too.

One of these experienced midwives will be able to spend time looking at your notes and history and she will discuss with you the pros and cons of induction of labour in your particular case. She may be able to advocate for you at any consultant meetings you have and help to make a personalised plan for you.

'Natural' methods of induction of labour

Evidence does not support the following methods for induction of labour:

- herbal supplements

- acupuncture

- homeopathy

- castor oil

- hot baths

- enemas

- sexual intercourse

While there is no evidence for sex helping to induce labour, it does seem logical that it might help. After all, skin-to-skin contact and orgasm raises oxytocin levels and the semen in the man's ejaculate has prostaglandins in it. So perhaps it's worth a try, though it's not recommended if your waters have released.

If you have had a straightforward pregnancy you may want to try nipple stimulation to attempt to help start off labour. When a baby nurses at the breast it produces a big hit of oxytocin and this is what nipple stimulation is trying to recreate. It takes a bit of persistence! Gently rub or roll your nipples and massage the darker area around your nipple (the areola) using your palm in a circular motion, firmly but gently. Do this for an hour, three times a day. Do 15 minutes on one breast, then switch to the other.

Conclusion

We are incredibly fortunate to have highly skilled doctors and midwives available to manage induction of labour and other interventions - and they can and do save lives. However, some feel that medical methods are overused, and that women are not given clear evidence relevant to their own specific situation to mull over beforehand. It is down to you to ask for this to be provided if wanted.

If you decide to accept induction of labour remember it is possible to have a very positive experience. You can still dim the lights, request as much assistance as possible to remain mobile while being monitored (like having the monitoring equipment set up whilst you're on the birth ball), and use your breathing and visualisations to keep things as relaxed as possible.

The website 'Tell me a good birth story' has many positive stories of induction of labour and there are some Facebook pages on this too.

The 'before birth' birth plan

When your due date comes... and goes... it can sometimes feel frustrating. It can also become irritating when well-meaning friends and family are constantly asking 'any news yet?'! After a few days of this, doubt and anxiety can creep in, potentially raising adrenalin levels, which is not the relaxed state you want to be in as you wait for your body and baby to tip into labour.

Thus it can be great to create a 'before birth' birth plan. Choose fourteen lovely things to do to keep you occupied and not sat at home just waiting for something to happen.

Here's a suggested plan:

Day 1: go out for dinner with your partner or a friend.

Day 2: if you'd enjoy it, go to an art gallery/local exhibition or book in for a one-day course.

Day 3: go to the cinema.

Day 4: book a relaxing pregnancy massage or maternity reflexology session.

Day 5: prepare some food such as pasta sauces, soups etc for the freezer in readiness for those early days of parenthood.

Day 6: do a yoga class then go for tea and cake ☺

Day 7: meet up with friends/family.

Day 8: plan a long, local walk with someone.

Day 9: get a haircut or have a facial.

Day 10: Have a pyjama day, relaxing and watching lots of comedy (laughter produces feel good hormones!).

Day 11: declutter the house, go through old photos, do all those odd jobs that will keep you occupied and you won't have time for when the baby arrives.

Day 12: watch some lovely birth videos, read positive birth stories, get a birth board ready.

Day 13: Go for a swim or to an aquanatal class.

Day 14: a gentle walk, a lovely takeaway with your partner and an early night (and perhaps some nipple stimulation!).

Further reading

Dr Sara Wickham - '*Inducing Labour – making informed decisions*'

http://www.ncbi.nlm.nih.gov/pubmedhealth/PMH0072755/)

Inducing Labour, NICE guidelines [cg70], NICE, 2008. Available at: https://www.nice.org.uk/guidance/cg70/ifp/chapter/What-is-induction-of-labour (Accessed August 2016)

https://www.nice.org.uk/guidance/cg70/chapter/introduction

https://www.nice.org.uk/guidance/CG70/chapter/1-Guidance#information-and-decision-making

NHS. http://www.nhs.uk/conditions/pregnancy-and-baby/pages/induction-labour.aspx

Kavanagh, J., Kelly, A.J. et al 'Breast stimulation for cervical ripening and induction of labour', *Cochrane Database of Systematic*

Reviews, 3.: CD003392, 2005. onlinelibrary.wiley.com (pdf file, Accessed May 2014)

http://www.babycentre.co.uk/a173/induced-labour

Association of Radical Midwives (ARM). Sweeping the Membranes. UK Midwifery Archives. Available at http://www.midwifery.org.uk (Accessed September 2016)

http://tellmeagoodbirthstory.com/

17

MONITORING

Labour can sometimes be stressful for a baby - a strong, healthy baby can cope well with this, but if a baby is unwell it may be harder for them meaning some babies need to be monitored continually. This is called electronic foetal monitoring (EFM). Your midwife may also use the term continuous cardiotocography (CTG) monitoring.

When might EFM be recommended? Some examples are -

- For multiple pregnancy and breech position.

- If a mother has high blood pressure.

- When the waters have been broken for over (18 - 24 hours) and broke before labour started.

- The baby has restricted growth concerns

- The woman's waters have meconium in them. Meconium is baby's first poo and can sometimes indicate the baby is distressed.

- Raised temperature, which may be pointing to an infection.

- Abnormal bleeding

- Previous caesarean birth

You may choose to decline EFM after discussing it with your caregiver, or you may feel after your questions have been answered fully that yes, you are happy to have this.

When you have EFM, two straps holding sensors are placed on your abdomen – one to measure contractions and the other to measure the baby's heart rate. This can make movement more difficult and you may be told you need to stay on the bed to be monitored – but you don't have to. You can still be active, but it may help if your partner holds on to the sensor during a surge to stop the reading being lost as you move about. Perhaps you can ask for an additional stretchy belt (which holds the monitor to you) to go on top of the other one, so you double up with belts. This may hold the sensor more firmly when you move about.

If you need to be monitored continually, ask if telemetry is available – this is wireless monitoring that will not interfere with your movement.

Unfortunately, EFM readings are not always accurately and reliably interpreted, and so your care thereafter should not be based on the readings alone. Other things should be taken into consideration, such as your baby's movements, how you are feeling, and other signs of complications.

Intermittent monitoring

This is done using a handheld device such as a pinnard stethoscope or sonicaid. Your midwife will find the right area on your abdomen and listen to the baby's heart beat. It doesn't usually affect movement or position. This is what will be used at a home birth and if your midwife suspects any problem she will swiftly transfer you into hospital and the baby will be monitored more closely.

During a water birth your midwife can use a waterproof sonicaid and you won't need to get out of the pool or lift your bump out of the water for her to listen in.

While continuous monitoring definitely has its place, it can have some down sides. As well as restricting a woman's mobility, and therefore her ability to cope with her labour well, it has been linked to an increased number of interventions in labour, including caesareans and assisted births, without any improvement in outcomes for babies.

NICE states 'Cardiotocography is not appropriate in the initial assessment of women at low risk of complications who are in labour. This is because it may lead to unnecessary interventions and does not provide any benefit to the baby.'

Further reading

https://www.nice.org.uk/guidance/QS105/chapter/Quality-statement-3-Cardiotocography-and-the-initial-assessment-of-a-woman-in-labour

https://www.nice.org.uk/guidance/qs105/chapter/Quality-statement-4-Stopping-cardiotocography

18

ASSISTED DELIVERY, STITCHES AND HEALING

Forceps and ventouse are instruments that are used to help a woman birth her baby and this is called an assisted birth. Assisted birth is offered if the mother is very tired or cannot feel to push, if labour is not progressing, if the baby is in distress or if the baby is in a less straightforward position.

Having an epidural and also induction of labour make an assisted birth more likely.

Having continuous support from someone you trust can reduce the chance of an assisted birth.

If an assisted birth is being suggested, you may like to ask if it is OK to have a little time, even a few minutes, alone with your partner to get your head around it all. Of course if it is a true emergency it will be obvious and that's a different situation, but if not, a few moments alone may, for example, give you some energy to perhaps change your position, galvanise some energy, or to mentally process the change in plan.

Before an assisted birth a woman will have either an injection to numb the perineum, or a spinal, or she may already have an epidural in place. Her bladder will be emptied using a catheter. She may need an episiotomy (a surgical cut to the perineum) in order to have an assisted birth. Any tears or episiotomies are repaired with dissolvable stitches. There is evidence that tissue that tears naturally heals better than a surgical cut, but an episiotomy may be appropriate at an instrumental delivery.

Sometimes a woman may have the procedure in theatre, and if the doctor is not reassured that the baby will be born safely by instrumental delivery, a caesarean birth may need to take place.

Forceps come in two halves. They carefully cradle the baby's head while he is in the birth canal and, when the woman has a contraction the doctor pulls at the same time, to help the baby out.

A ventouse is a small cap that is sometimes attached to a suction pump. The small cap fits onto the baby's head and stays attached with suction. The ventouse is then pulled to help the baby be born as the mother pushes.

Sometimes the baby's head may be bruised, cut or misshapen following an assisted birth, but healing is usually straightforward and any marks normally disappear after 24–48 hours.

Verbal consent is required before either of these procedures takes place. It should always be explained to you why an intervention needs to take place.

Active management of the third stage is recommended after an instrumental birth.

Healing after stitches or a tear

- Research states that being mobile helps as this increases the blood flow to the perineum

- You may find bathing in warm water and/or using a Valley cushion (a specially designed inflatable cushion to make sitting down more comfortable) may help.

- Regular pain killers can help ease discomfort – your midwife will be able to advise which are safe to take if you are breastfeeding.

- If you find you're still very uncomfortable after a week or so, speak with your midwife, health visitor or GP and don't suffer in silence. It could be that you have an infection which will make things more painful and slower to heal.

You might want to try the following suggestions during the healing period as well:

- You can pour water over your perineum whilst you wee, if you are concerned about a stinging sensation – or wee in the shower or just before you get out of the bath. Try leaning forward when weeing if you have had an episiotomy.

- After going to the toilet pour a jug of warm water over your perineum to rinse it rather than wiping with toilet tissue, then gently dab the area to dry it.

- If you feel constipated and a high-fibre diet and staying hydrated has not helped, ask your midwife or GP about suitable, gentle laxatives.

- The moment you feel the urge to open your bowels take action right away and sit on the toilet. You can use the second stage breathing – no hard pushing required here either!

- It sounds obvious but do remember to wipe front to back, away from your vagina, to make sure your stitches remain clean.

- Place an ice-pack or ice-cubes, wrapped in a cloth, to relieve discomfort.

- Restart your pelvic floor exercises as soon as you can after birth. They enhance blood circulation, and aid the healing process.

- Ask for a referral to a specialist women's-health physiotherapist if you feel you would benefit from this.

- When you feel ready you could attend a postnatal pilates class with a well qualified instructor to help with your core strength. Often there are day time classes where you can bring your baby along with you.

Further reading

https://www.rcog.org.uk/globalassets/documents/patients/patient-information-leaflets/pregnancy/pi-an-assisted-vaginal-birth-ventouse-or-forceps.pdf

http://mobile.oaaformothers.info/

19

PERINEAL MASSAGE

The perineum is the area between the anus (back passage) and the bottom edge of the vulva. During labour it gets stretched and becomes very thin. This is usual and helps bring about a powerful surge of oxytocin to aid your baby's birth.

Sometimes the perineum may tear during birth, and massaging the area daily from around 36 weeks may reduce the likelihood of perineal trauma as it may help this tissue expand more easily during birth.

If a woman has practised perineal massage antenatally, she may feel less anxious as she knows she has spent time and effort gently and gradually stretching the perineum. She will be familiar with the stretched feeling she will feel as her baby's head is crowning and will not be frightened by it. Therefore she will be able to relax into this stage, which may help prevent tearing.

How to carry out perineal massage

- Get comfortable, lying against some pillows on the bed, with your legs bent at the knees so you or your partner can reach your perineum. You can also try laying on your side and reaching the perineum from underneath your bottom.

- Some women prefer to try perineal massage after they have had a bath and are feeling relaxed.

- Massage a lubricant such as a vegetable based oil or any carrier oil (no need to buy a special perineal massage oil - unless you want to) into the skin of the perineum.

- Then place your clean thumb (with a short nail) around 3-4cm (or roughly up to the thumb's first knuckle) inside your vagina and press downwards towards the anus.

- Move to each side in a U-shaped stretching movement. This may give a tingling/burning sensation.

- Hold the stretch for 30-60 seconds then release.

- Some find it hard to reach the perineum, in which case your partner can do it for you.

- Do not do perineal massage if you have vaginal herpes, thrush or any other vaginal infection

Whilst it might not be the most comfortable of things to do, it should not be painful, if you feel pain stop and try again another time. If you continue to feel pain discuss this with your midwife.

Further reading

http://onlinelibrary.wiley.com/doi/10.1002/14651858.CD005
123.pub3/abstract;jsessionid=43415DBAB9C362347431609A
9C8AAA65.f03t04

20

CAESAREAN BIRTH

A caesarean birth (also known as caesarean section or c-section) is an operation where the baby is born via an incision in the lower abdomen and uterus. Caesareans can be either planned or unplanned (taking place during labour).

Planned caesareans are usually carried out after 39 weeks unless there is a medical reason to do it sooner. Your date may change if another woman requires a caesarean and her needs are more pressing than yours. If appropriate, you may be able to negotiate waiting until you go into labour.

 Most women recover well after a caesarean birth, though there are risks associated with all surgery, and it will take longer to get 'back to normal' afterwards.

Currently in the UK, caesarean birth is not recommended unless there is a medical reason that makes it necessary. If a woman is being refused a caesarean for non-medical reasons guidance states she should be referred on to another obstetrician or hospital.

For some women it is recommended that they give birth via caesarean. Reasons could include:

- Placental issues such as placenta praevia (when the placenta covers the outlet) or placental abruption (when the placenta starts to come away from the uterus wall).

- Medical issues such as raised blood pressure (pre-eclampsia).

- Your baby's position – if your baby is lying transverse or oblique (across) or breech (although some women choose to opt for a vaginal breech birth).

- If your baby is in a breech position doctors may offer to try to turn your baby into a head down position using pressure on your abdomen. This procedure is called an ECV (External Cephalic Version) and is usually offered at around 36 or so weeks of pregnancy. It has about a 50% success rate. Some babies just turn back as perhaps this is the right position for them! If your baby is in a breech position ask your midwife about moxibustion – a type of acupuncture which may be effective between 34-36 weeks of pregnancy.

- Multiple pregnancy – although some women have vaginal twin births.

- If labour is not progressing and the woman agrees to a caesarean for this.

- Severe growth restriction

Some women are anxious about giving birth vaginally, for a variety of reasons including having a fear of childbirth (tokophobia). Others are worried their partner may miss the birth as he or she will be away when they are due.

If you have concerns about your birth you can discuss this with your midwife who may offer to refer you on to perinatal mental health specialist to talk through this. If a woman continues to ask for a caesarean birth it should be performed.

What are the risks for caesarean birth?

All surgery carries risks and we all view risk differently. Risk is very personal and our feelings about it can be dependent on past experiences and how we view things.

If a woman is healthy and well the risks are reduced. The main risks of giving birth by caesarean are:

- Wound infection – this is common. It can take some time for the wound to heal, perhaps several weeks.

- Blood clots developing in the legs – which may travel up into the lungs. To help try to prevent this compression stockings are usually issued and sometimes blood thinning injections.

- Heavy bleeding.

- Damage to internal organs such as the bladder or bowel

- Babies born by caesarean may need assistance with breathing or require time in the special care baby unit.

- Babies are at a small risk of being cut during the procedure (1–2 in 100), though this is usually not deep and heals well.

- Any risks that the anaesthetic used may bring.

A first caesarean is usually a relatively simple operation, but subsequent caesareans are not so predictable, due to the scar tissue that remains from the previous surgery. If a woman has had a caesarean for her first baby (or subsequent babies) she can choose to have a vaginal birth next time if she wishes and this is called a VBAC (Vaginal Birth After Caesarean).

What happens during a caesarean?

The exact procedure can vary from hospital to hospital.

- The woman needs to read and sign a consent form before the operation.

- She will need to put on a hospital gown, remove any jewellery, contact lenses and sometimes she is asked to remove nail polish (so the nail bed can be viewed easily to check oxygen blood levels) and her bikini area may be shaved in theatre.

- If the caesarean section is not an emergency usually a she receives a regional anaesthetic, which can be given via an epidural if one is already in place, or by spinal, which is similar to an epidural but quicker acting. The drugs given mean she will not feel any pain, but she will feel some sensation, like a tugging, which is normal. She will be awake for her baby's birth.

- Sometimes a woman has the procedure under a general anaesthetic and in these cases partners cannot come into the theatre.

There are lots of people present at a caesarean birth, usually at least 8 or more, so don't be alarmed when you see the room fill up as this is normal.

As a rough guide, your baby will be born within around the first five minutes and the rest of the operation takes around 45 minutes to an hour, longer for multiple births.

The placenta is removed during the procedure. If you want to have delayed cord clamping this usually needs to be discussed in advance of the birth.

You can hold your baby right away providing they do not require any medical attention. Some mothers choose to breastfeed while in theatre, others prefer to wait until they are in the recovery room.

Lots and lots of skin to skin with the baby after birth is always good and will also help the mother's milk 'come in' if she's planning on breastfeeding. Ask your midwife for help with holding positions that won't touch or knock your lower abdomen.

Parent Centred/Natural Approach to Caesarean Birth

If for whatever reason you are going to give birth via caesarean if of interest, you can ask about a natural caesarean. The following points may or may not be an option and is something it would ideally be best to talk through in advance if at all possible.

During a natural caesarean once the incision has been made, the baby partially emerges by himself from the uterus, which can take around four minutes. The curtain is removed or lowered so the mother can see her baby being born rather than the doctor doing this speedily. As the baby emerges, the parents can discover the sex themselves. He is then placed onto his mother for immediate skin to skin. Being born this way may lower the chance of the baby having respiratory problems which can sometime occur with the traditional method.

What is recovery like after a caesarean?

The mother is transferred to a postnatal ward where she will stay from between 24 hours to 1 - 3 days, depending on her specific situation. She often feels uncomfortable for the first 2-3 days and strong painkillers are offered. It gets easier over time with full recovery time varying from woman to woman. Keep on top of the timings of your aftercare medication so the relief is consistent.

Keeping mobile helps with managing any pain or discomfort. Try to stand up straight and gently change your position from time to time.

The wound can feel sore for a few weeks after the operation.

Some women suffer with trapped wind pain or difficulty urinating – talk to your midwife if this happens.

Take a few deep breaths every hour to clear your lungs and when coughing, sneezing or laughing, bend your legs or hold a pillow over your tummy to help with discomfort.

You should be given some information on gentle exercises to do – ask for this if you have not.

As with after any birth it is important to take it easy and to not be in a rush to get back to normal. If you had your appendix out or any other operation for example would you rush back to work? We tend to expect mothers to get back to normal (whatever 'normal' is!) quickly after birth, including a caesarean birth, which puts pressure on her.

Avoid strenuous exercise and driving for around 6 weeks or (just like you would after any operation!). Check with your GP and car insurance if you want to drive sooner than this. You can always ask about these things at your 6-week GP check, which is an appointment to see how you and your baby are doing.

If a woman has had an unplanned caesarean she may feel mixed emotions and question why things did not go as she planned and hoped for. Women can arrange to talk through their birth with a midwife to get answers and explanations, which may help them feel at peace with what happened and why. This service is available for all women, regardless of what type of birth they had – you just need to request it.

In the UK it's fairly standard for partners to get two weeks' leave from work after their baby's birth. Who can you call upon after this time to help you with things, or who can pop by to support and nurture you and maybe take over a bit so you can rest?

Further reading

https://www.rcog.org.uk/globalassets/documents/patients/patient-information-leaflets/pregnancy/pi-choosing-to-have-a-c-section.pdf

NHS Choices – Caesarean section:

www.nhs.uk/Conditions/Caesarean-section/Pages/Introduction.aspx

NICE guideline on caesarean section:

www.nice.org.uk/guidance/cg132/informationforpublic

http://www.caesarean.org.uk/

NHS Maternity Statistics – England, 2014-2015, Health & Social Care Information Centre, (HSCIC), 2016.

http://www.caesarean.org.uk/

https://www.nct.org.uk/birth/what-happens-during-elective-or-emergency-caesarean-section

21

BIRTH PLANS / BIRTH PREFERENCES

You don't have to write a birth plan, but many people choose to. You can follow a template such as the NHS one which is available online, or create your own. Your midwife may give you one or a template may be in your handheld notes.

It can be helpful to write your birth preferences sheet with your birth partner so he or she is aware of your hopes and wishes. During the active phase of labour when surges are at their most powerful you may not want to talk, so if your partner is aware of you want it can help you to focus only on yourself.

Some may say 'What's the point of writing a birth plan, it all goes out the window anyway?' – but why would you not plan for and think about what you might like to happen during the biggest, most important thing you will ever do?

Yes, birth can be unpredictable, which is why being very flexible and planning for every eventuality can be useful. Once you have written your birth plan, put aside any concerns and spend time and effort focusing on the birth you want and not on the 'what ifs'. If the 'what ifs' happen not only will you have

highly skilled carers with you to help, but you
prepared for them and thought about what you wc
that situation, which afterwards can help you feel more au
peace with how things went.

Ideas to think about for your birth plan

If you have practised using hypnobirthing you can put a short
section at the front of the birth plan mentioning this.

You can then add in some or all of the following, as you see fit.
Some of these suggestions might not appeal to you in which
case you can just omit them.

Using bullet points and keeping it to one page is helpful. Bring
along several copies and your birth partner can ensure it gets
read. In the unlikely event that you feel it is not being taken
seriously request to change midwife! No one should be making
light of your hopes and wishes.

- Where possible, I would be very grateful if you would
  direct any questions to my birth partner initially.

- If mother and baby are doing well we'd prefer to allow
  our birth to take its time.

- I would like a dimly-lit, quiet environment and want to
  give birth at home/on the midwife-led unit/on the
  labour ward.

- Please don't offer me pain relief, if this is something I
  would like I will ask for it at the time. *OR*, my pain

relief options are, in order of preference (list your preferences).

- I would like to be encouraged to keep gently active and use equipment like a birth ball, birth stool or bean bags.

- In the absence of a medical emergency, please do not offer coached pushing at the second stage. I want to follow my body's lead to birth my baby.

- I would/would not like student midwives or doctors in with me.

- I would not like any vaginal examinations (remember you can always change your mind about this, or anything else!) OR, I would like just one initial assessment, OR I am happy to have regular examinations. Perhaps you'd like to ask that your partner gets told how dilated you are so they relay this information to you in their encouraging words. Or rather than be told how many centimetres you are dilated, instead be informed whether you are progressing well, or not.

- I would like to try the birth pool.

- If my baby's heart rate is reassuring and if it is appropriate, I would like to be intermittently monitored so I can move freely.

- I would prefer not to be disturbed when in active labour – please feel free to do any routine checks without asking for my permission.

- I would like to be the first one to touch my baby and lift my baby up to me myself/for my partner to do this.

- I would like my baby lifted straight on to me/to have skin-to-skin right away or, I would like a few minutes before holding my baby.

- If there is no medical emergency, we'd like weighing and measuring to wait so we can enjoy our first moments together as a family.

- I would like a physiological third stage or I would like active management of the third stage. My partner would / would not like to cut the cord. Or, I would like to cut the cord.

- I would like help with breastfeeding right away/I am not planning on breastfeeding.

- We would like/not like our baby to have Vitamin K (injection or orally?).

- If my baby needs to be moved away from me I would like my partner to stay with him/her.

In the event of an induction of labour, I would like:

- If appropriate during the induction process, to have some time to walk about after having my waters broken to see if things get going by themselves before starting the syntocinon.

- To keep as active as possible and not be on the bed.

any monitoring set up whilst I'm on the birth
remain active.

he lights low and interruption to a minimum.

- To try without an epidural *OR* I would like an epidural.

- If my baby has to go to SCBU (special care baby unit), I want my partner to stay with him/her.

In the event of an unplanned caesarean birth, if possible, I would like:

- Uninterrupted skin-to-skin right away.

- To find out our baby's gender ourselves.

- To have the curtain lowered at the time of birth so I can see my baby being born.

- To have our own music played if there is time for this.

- To bring our camera/phone in for first pictures.

- If my baby has to go to SCBU (special care baby unit), I want my partner to stay with him/her.

Thank you very much for taking care of me during my baby's birth!

A reminder of things to consider in advance

- Whether or not you will consent to a membranes' sweep.

- Your thoughts on your 'due date' – do you need to book in a chat with someone senior to personalise your plans?

- Do you need to think about a second birth partner/doula?

- Monitoring – what options are available to you?

- Whether or not you agree to having your waters broken during labour – this may only shave around an hour off your labour, but it will make the surges feel stronger and more intense.

- A quiet, dimly-lit environment where you will feel safe – remember external dictates internal and labour progresses best when you feel safe, secure and not unduly interrupted.

- Keeping active and off the bed – if you practice your positions in advance you are more likely to use them on the day.

Further reading:

Fletcher, S. Mindful Hypnobirthing Hypnosis and Mindfulness Techniques for a Calm and Confident Birth

Graves, K. The Hypnobirthing Book

I'M EXPECTING A BABY

22

HEALING AND RESTING AFTER BIRTH

Many women are in such a rush to get back to normal after birth that the importance of a period of rest and nurturing following birth is overlooked. Whatever type of birth you have had, you need time to mentally adjust to becoming a mother, as well as time to physical healing. Therefore it is great to make a postnatal plan. While the birth is of course very important, so is your recovery.

Who can you call upon to support you once your baby is here? What can you do now to help prepare for the crazy, chaotic early days of parenthood?

Below are some ideas for you to consider.

Visitors

- How do you feel about visitors after the birth? Would you prefer to have some time alone with your baby, just you and your partner, before welcoming visitors? Or are you happy to have visitors right away?

- Would you prefer to have everyone over on a set day, at a set time? How about asking them all to bring a dish so you can eat together. Get some paper plates/cups and plastic cutlery so you're not left with the washing up after they go!

- How about limiting visiting time? You could make it after lunch so it is clear that you are not providing a meal. Offer visiting from, say, 2–4pm – making it clear that after this you need to rest.

- How useful will your visitors be? If they are the type who would nurture you by bringing food and some shopping and being mindful to leave when you're tired then great.

- If you are planning on breastfeeding it can be easier to sit in bed with your top off spending time getting to grips with it, or you may just want lots of bonding skin to skin with your baby – you may not feel comfortable doing this with relatives sitting opposite you!

Your baby may be over-stimulated by the inevitable game of 'pass the baby', and any strong perfumes or aftershaves people are wearing. Lying down in a dimly-lit room and having skin-to-skin can help to calm your baby. All they want is you, after all.

Bleeding after birth

Postnatal bleeding (lochia) is healthy and normal following any type of birth – both vaginal and caesarean – and is not painful though some mothers experience after pains when breastfeeding (less so with a first baby). If you are in pain speak to your midwife.

Lochia blood loss from the placental site (womb) continues until the lining is renewed. It can last up to 6 weeks, but it won't be heavy for all that time and many women find it gradually reduces and stops by around 2 weeks after the birth.

Stock up on around 4 packs of maternity pads – do not use tampons. For the first day the blood loss is usually bright red and may have clots in it. If you are passing large clots, lots of clots or soaking through sanitary pads mention this to your midwife. Expect to change your pad around every couple of hours in the first few days.

Just like a period does, the blood loss will change colour from red to a brown colour to a pinky mucous loss, becoming less over the first 10 days. For some women it peters out more quickly than for others. Once the loss has lessened you can use a panty liner rather than big, bulky maternity pads.

Stock up on big, comfy knickers – there is no need to buy paper ones unless you want to.

Retained placenta

Sometimes a fragment of placenta may be left behind inside the uterus, which can cause problems and needs to be dealt with quickly. If you experience any of the following symptoms, go to your doctor or speak to your midwife.

- heavy bleeding

- cramping

- foul-smelling vaginal discharge

- fever

- a lack of breastmilk

Also contact your doctor if you have prolonged, heavy bleeding in the days or weeks following your baby's birth. Seek medical help if your blood flow peters off, then suddenly becomes very heavy again.

Pain relief after birth

Take advice from a qualified healthcare professional as to what types of pain killers are safe for you as women's circumstances are varied.

Breastfeeding

It can sometimes take a while for you and your baby to get the hang of breastfeeding. If you find it a struggle seek help through the NCT Breastfeeding Helpline on 0300 330 0771 (8am - midnight, 7 days a week) or via a drop in session/a breastfeeding cafe. There are useful websites and phone numbers on this at the end of the book.

Sex life

It is of course usual for your sex drive to take a back seat after birth! Adjusting to your new role and giving your body time to heal is important. Some women feel ready sooner than others, with some women preferring to wait until their 6-week check with the GP - or longer.

While you're exclusively breastfeeding, levels of oestrogen stay low to prevent you ovulating and falling pregnant, but this should *not* be relied on as contraception. At your 6-week GP check your doctor will discuss safe methods of contraception, which may be different from your previous methods – for example, certain types of the pill may not be suitable if you are breastfeeding.

Emotions

Some parents feel a huge rush of love when they meet their baby for the first time, while for others it may take a little longer. Try not to worry if you don't feel strong love straight away. Many things can affect this, including how you feel your birth went. Go easy on yourself and give yourself time.

It is normal for mothers to feel emotional, teary and overwhelmed after birth, and around 80 per cent of mothers experience the so-called 'baby blues'. No one really knows exactly what causes baby blues, but it is not an illness and should pass by the time your baby is around 10 days old (usually within 48 hours or so). Symptoms include feeling irrational, teary, irritable, anxious or 'touchy'.

Sometimes parents feel depressed after the birth of their baby — this can affect both mothers and fathers and is called postnatal depression. Depression can be made worse by emotional and stressful events and what support a person has available has a huge affect on how they feel they can cope, along with disturbed sleep, possibly how the birth went, relationship issues, money pressures and so on.

The sooner you or your partner's feelings are talked through the better — recovery may be slower for some than others, but it will happen, and there is a lot of help out there (information on sources of help can be found at the end of the book).

- Share your feelings with people you trust and who will not judge you. It could be a health visitor, a friend or a counsellor.

- Talking to other mums and dads can be very reassuring, or those who have experienced postnatal depression before. There may be a local meet-up near you.

- Try to get time away from your baby; even an hour here and there can make a difference. You are important too!

- Take some exercise each day, such as a walk with your baby or perhaps doing a postnatal pilates or yoga class. Exercise has a positive effect on mood.

- Maintain a healthy diet: eating badly or skipping meals can make you feel tired and irritable, try to eat simple and nutritious meals. There is some evidence that foods rich in omega-3 oils can help with depression.

- Accept help and support from family and friends. Is there anyone you trust who could take your baby for a walk for an hour or so whilst you sleep?

- Speak to your GP about having a blood test to check iron levels, etc.

- Give yourself time to adjust to parenthood.

Postpartum psychosis

Postpartum psychosis (also known as puerperal psychosis) is a serious mental illness which always requires psychiatric treatment and a stay in hospital. It only affects the mother and is rare, affecting around one or two mothers in every 1,000, and most commonly occurs in the first month after having a baby (usually within the few days or so).

The main symptoms of puerperal psychosis are delusions, hallucinations, confused thoughts and a lack of self-awareness. In very severe cases, a woman may try to harm her baby and/or herself, and medical help is required immediately and in the first instance via Accident & Emergency (A&E) who will then refer on for help with care going forward. Usually after medication a woman feels a lot better quite quickly, though full recovery will likely take some time.

Nutrition

Even though your baby may sleep up to 16 hours a day, it is still surprisingly hard to fit in preparing and eating food –

unless you have planned in advance or have friends and family close by to help!

You can prepare for this before the birth. If you are making pasta sauce, cook for six instead of two and freeze four portions. Separate food into small glass dishes before freezing them, that way they can go directly into the oven without having to be defrosted first. Or make a vat of soup and bag and freeze several portions. Set up an internet shop with a supermarket and ask visitors to bring supplies (or even better a meal!).

Exercise

Unless you exercised regularly before the birth of your baby, it's usually best to start slowly and wait until your 6-week postnatal check with your GP who can advise you before starting a serious exercise regime again. This will be longer if you have had a caesarean birth, possibly 3 – 6 months.

High-impact exercise is not advised until at least 3 months after birth and is would be a good idea to talk to a trained professional about this first. Something like swimming (once postnatal bleeding has ceased), yoga or a postnatal pilates class would be great, as would getting out for some fresh air with your baby once a day for your all important mental health.

Final words

I hope this book has given you food for thought and faith in your incredible body and powerful mind. And I hope the suggested ideas for birth partners serve you well.

If you are being told 'you're not allowed to...' or 'you have to...' this is a sign that you need to ask questions! Always take the time to do your own research and ensure you are getting personalised care.

Whilst birth is unpredictable, there is so much you can do to make it positive even down to changing the labour ward room around.

Invest time and effort into practising the hypnobirthing and breathing techniques, starting daily practise as early as you can.

Consider an in depth antenatal course and/or a hypnobirthing course if you are open to this, attend a good pregnancy yoga class, work on your mindset by reading as much birth positivity as possible and block out all negativity.

Remember the BRAIN acronym – if you ask, there is usually always time for someone to take the time to explain things to you and possible another option available which hadn't been mentioned. You deserve clear explanations on the benefits and risks of things being offered to you, and being pointed to evidence that backs this up.

For the women reading this book - you were built to do this and you are truly amazing.

Wishing you all the very best for birth and beyond!

Useful websites, phone numbers & authors

For general pregnancy &/or postnatal topics:

www.nct.org.uk

www.kickscount.org.uk

For information and statistics on your particular hospital & for general information:

www.which.co.uk/birth-choice/

Birth Research & information

www.sarawickham.com

www.aims.org.uk

www.evidencebasedbirth.com

www.midwifethinking.com

Your rights in birth/support with your choices

www.birthrights.org.uk

www.aims.org.uk

PALS – the Patient Advisory & Liaison Service (based at each UK Hospital)

Positive Birth Support:

www.positivebirthmovement.org

www.tellmeagoodbirthstory.com

Evidence based guidelines for the UK:

www.nice.org.uk

https://www.nice.org.uk/guidance/cg190?unlid=46050102020
163113029

Breastfeeding help:
https://www.nct.org.uk/parenting/breastfeeding-concerns
NCT Breastfeeding line – 0300 330 0770 (8am – midnight, every day)

Breastfeeding Network Supporter line – 08444 412 4664
(9.30am – 9.30pm every day)
La Leche League 0845 120 2918

Independent Midwives & Doulas:
www.imuk.org.uk

Mental Health/Pre & Postnatal Depression support:
www.pandasfoundation.org.uk

Books - there are so many fantastic books out there (some have been mentioned within the chapters), but here are a few others well worth reading:

Grantly Dick-Read - Childbirth without Fear
Ina May Gaskin – Ina May's Guide to Childbirth
Mark Harris – Men, Love & Birth
Susanna Heli – Confident Birth
Milli Hill – Positive Birth Book
Maggie Howell – Effective Birth Preparation
All the Dr Sara Wickham and Association for Improvement in Maternity Services (AIMS) books relevant to you!

I'M EXPECTING A BABY

17470538R00140

Printed in Great Britain
by Amazon